AIDS

WHAT THE GOVERNMENT ISN'T TELLING YOU

LORRAINE DAY, M.D.

ROCKFORD PRESS
PALM DESERT, CALIFORNIA

Rockford Press
44-489 Town Center Way, Suite D-412
Palm Desert, CA 92260

Library of Congress Catalog Card Number 91-75346
ISBN 0-9630940-0-9

First Rockford Press printing September 1991

10 9 8 7 6 5 4 3 2

Printed in the U.S.A.

In memory of my father, John Osborn,
whose honesty, integrity and love
have been my guiding light.

Preface

The seeds of this book were planted in my childhood by my father who frequently listened to my pleas to "do what all the other kids are doing." He would then respond, "Herd instinct; why do you want to do what the herd is doing? Why don't you decide what's right and stand on your own two feet!" While I was growing up, both my father and mother instilled in my brother and me the importance of honesty and integrity. "Don't ever compromise your principles for personal, financial or political gain," they told us again and again.

As a young orthopedic surgeon and assistant professor at the University of California, San Francisco and San Francisco General Hospital, my days were filled with many duties, including teaching medical students and resident doctors in training, operating on patients and caring for them both in and out of the hospital. Nearly everyone I worked with was honest and straight-forward.

As I moved up the ladder and interacted with the leaders of both the hospital and the university I was perplexed, saddened and even repulsed to perceive how much these leaders had compromised the principles they must have had at some earlier time. For example, during one private meeting, the University Dean informed me I was "too prickly" in standing for principles. "But what do you want me to do," I asked, "sell my soul?" His response was astonishing to me and forced me to understand the enormity of the "integrity" problem in our medical institutions. He placed his chin in his hand and looked me squarely in the eye; "Sooner or later everyone sells his soul," said this physician, whom heretofore I had admired.

Virtually every medical and governmental agency I dealt with had a hidden agenda, mainly political, that kept them from handling the AIDS epidemic according to well-established public health guidelines. For a long time I was confused, unable to understand why no one seemed interested in hearing the truth, much less publicizing it and acting on it.

Everyone was so busy behaving in the "politically correct" mode, a mode often necessary to keep one's job, that creative and imaginative political rationalizations were constructed to explain abominable committee decisions—decisions that often led to loss of life.

On October 2, 1987, when I suddenly realized that the AIDS epidemic was much more ominous than I had been told, I began working privately, not publicly, through hospital channels and medical committees to inject some common sense into the proposed rules and regulations. In the early days of my involvement, never once did I even think of "going public" with my information. But when I found that my colleagues were saying one thing privately in committees and another thing to the press and the public, I decided that the public had a right to know the truth. So anytime I was approached by the media, I agreed to speak.

The ostracism that followed was unpleasant, and the threats of bodily harm that have been directed at those who speak out on this issue have been worrisome. But when I tried to back away, my father's influence, like a recording, began to play in my conscience. "Don't do what the herd does. Decide what's right and stand on your own two feet."

Over the past several years, I have been very critical of those in government and in the medical establishment who lack the courage to speak the truth about AIDS. If I chose to remain silent because of pressures and threats that have come not only from special interest groups but from well established institutions of our country, I would be reacting in the same manner as those I have criticized.

I made the decision to tell what I know for the safety of the unsuspecting public, for the safety of my fellow health care workers who are taking far greater risks than the government is admitting, and for my children and the children of other concerned parents who understand that this disease does not discriminate. It can infect anyone.

There have been many who have supported my efforts: my orthopedic surgery residents, who for years have been my extended family; my office staff at San Francisco General Hospital including Mr. Wiley Herring, my administrative analyst, whose advice was often of critical importance and whose perception of events was right on target. His loyalty, friendship and protectiveness sustained me through some very difficult and uncomfortable times.

Many thanks and much gratitude to my assistant, Karlene Wach, who for some period of time, between many months and eternity, was physically attached, it seems, to her computer and this manuscript, in-putting change after change, draft after draft, with her characteristic cheerfulness and good humor with only an occasional menacing scream of exasperation followed by a barely audible threat of suicide if I changed one more word.

Also, I have been buoyed by the hundreds of letters of support I have received from doctors throughout the country, particularly my fellow orthopedic surgeons, who knew me before I became involved in this issue, and vouched that I was not a "nut" as the journalists so often portrayed me. And I have been sustained by the millions of Americans who have the common sense to question what they're being told by the government and the medical establishment. To them, it just doesn't make sense.

To all of you who read this book and realize that our leaders are playing a deadly game with our lives and the lives of our children, I challenge you to get organized and make your voices heard.

Individuals can make a difference. Individuals are the only ones who make a difference. There are no statues to committees!

L.D.

September 1991

Contents

1

Don't Believe the "Experts"

This is a book that's written from the heart, mind, creed and conscience of one lone physician who has watched the appalling power ploys surrounding AIDS. These power ploys, as presently permitted, make for bad medicine.

AIDS is the most politicized disease mankind has ever known. Special interest groups have helped subvert the health care policies we have in place—good policies that should apply to all diseases.

I am an American orthopedic trauma surgeon—living and working in San Francisco, one of the two AIDS capitols in the Western world.

I feel deeply about AIDS and what it will do to our future. Were I to choose a cause, however, it probably would not be AIDS.

It has become a cause for me entirely by default, because when I stand in the operating room, I stand in human blood.

There is blood everywhere—in my shoes, on my sleeves, and all over the floor. There is blood on every instrument and power tool I use. Human blood soaks through my gown and through my underwear. It settles on my abdominal skin. It trickles down my forearms. It seeps between my toes.

That blood is potentially as deadly as somebody's pistol held to my temple. I don't know who will trigger it. I'm not allowed to know.

I will give you unnerving facts regarding AIDS that research is unraveling, and "facts" I can only suspect, that await serious, unbiased research to verify or banish.

This is a volume made of glimpses and vignettes, of newspaper reports and anecdotal interviews. Much more importantly, this book cites crucial, documented research buried in the professional literature—research that the man in the street, the nurse on the ward and the parent with a child in the playground must know.

I will paint you a kaleidoscope of horror.

Although undoubtedly some people will see this book as ammunition, it's neither a vehicle meant for reactionary thought nor a means, conversely, of comforting my gay friends and foes, my colleagues and *politicos.*

And it decidedly is not a book that's cowardly.

This book is meant as an arrow. The target is your common sense.

Some things regarding AIDS cry out to be said in clear, crisp language by someone with credentials. I'd like to cite mine here.

I have a medical degree and am a specialist in orthopedic surgery. In addition, I have done much work towards my Ph.D. in cell biology. I have to my credit some fifteen years of practice in the operating room as a staff member of one of the outstanding trauma hospitals in the country.

I lecture world-wide and testify at crucial trials involving ground-breaking issues pertaining to the AIDS virus. For many years, I was on the full-time faculty as an associate professor and vice chairman of the Department of Orthopedic Surgery at the University of California, San Francisco.

I have been a member of the AIDS Committee of San Francisco General Hospital and the University of California, San Francisco. I am a member of the AIDS Task Force of the American Academy of Orthopedic Surgeons.

For five years, I was Chief of the Orthopedic Surgery Service at San Francisco General Hospital, the only trauma hospital in that city.

Although I haven't done a survey and have no stake in setting professional records, I believe that I have performed surgery on as many HIV-infected patients as anyone else in the country. If there's a stretcher with a bleeding patient at San Francisco General, the chance of that patient having AIDS is very high indeed.

Avoiding jargon and excessive footnotes, and writing in language a lay person can understand, I aim this book at that mysterious place within my readers where rationality resides, and where decency and sanity, combined with a healthy anger, will trigger appropriate action.

With credit to a San Franciscan journalist, Randy Shilts, a well-known homosexual who first thought up the word, this book will be, in essence, not about AIDS so much as about *AIDSpeak.*

AIDSpeak, stripped down to its essentials, sells you that old line of the Depression era that warns "the only thing you have to fear is fear itself."

Alas, how false!

This naive attitude, at present provides the shadow troops

for AIDS. It has attached itself to AIDS—the ugliest disease that I have ever seen, and the first massively and systematically politicized disease that has been falsified, misrepresented, and then whitewashed to the public: We as Americans had better learn to render these forces powerless—and fast.

This book is a weapon that may well be hurled against me rather than by me. I'd like to state up front, not that it matters much, that it is not meant to fan the flames of prejudice. I'd like to go on record here and now that I am not against homosexuals.

I'd like to keep them alive. I'd like to see them keep themselves alive. And although some of my closest friends are homosexual—regrettably, some homosexuals have become my fiercest enemies.

This book is about the fundamental duty of gays, as well as straights, to protect themselves and to protect loved ones against AIDSpeak as much as against the lethal virus itself.

AIDSpeak, if allowed to indoctrinate you, will blur your fear of the virus.

You can't afford *not* to have fear. You must have fear. You must.

You can't afford to let somebody else's political, social or sexual agenda foist a deadly virus on you unsuspectingly, a microbe that kills every body it invades.

How did I manage to acquire this image of warmongering?

I guess because I found myself all of a sudden in the trenches, a foot soldier in a war nobody bothered to define or declare and, therefore, nobody took the trouble to wage with winning strategies.

Day after day, week after week, I stood in killer blood up to my ankles, while people I had heretofore respected as my colleagues ridiculed my "silly" fear and called me some pretty unflattering names.

Laymen do not realize that even in the medical profession, great ignorance exists among non-surgeons about what goes on during surgery. It is possible to go through medical school and never once step physically into an operating room, much less do any kind of surgery. It is as if those of us who make a living with a scalpel and those who are non-surgical live on two different planets.

I speak specifically about that huge, unwieldy bureaucracy that deals with infectious diseases. In our present academic atmosphere, controlled by grants and, hence, by politics that often are special interest politics, it is all too advantageous for someone with a yen for recognition and advancement to publish a "scientific" article that toes the party line.

The present party line in hospitals is this: AIDS is being neatly kept in check with "universal precautions," namely gloves, gowns and goggles.

I am here to say it is not. AIDS remains dangerously on the loose.

Orthopedic surgery means doing heavy-duty work such as a carpenter might do. I work on bone. I work with power tools on human bodies that harbor the most deadly virus this globe has seen since the Middle Ages, maybe ever.

I cut. I drill. I saw. Sometimes I chop away at hard bone much like a woodcutter might chop away at a tree trunk. There are splinters. There are splashes. There are rivers of red flowing down my gown, dripping on my legs, my feet, and the floor.

I receive patients from emergency, who have been severely injured in car crashes, in accidents, who have fallen out of windows, who have been shot with machine guns in gang wars, who have bone fragments protruding through their flesh as sharp as splinters from a crystal glass that has been smashed against a fireplace. These fragments will cut through my gloves.

I get cut often, and over time, I have received scores of needlesticks. I get injured on equipment, not because I am clumsy but because it is the nature of my work.

If it's an AIDS-infected patient on whom I have to work, I am in mortal danger of being killed by the one whose life I am trying to save.

Even during routine surgery such as a hip replacement, I stand within a fine red mist of human blood. My power drill makes aerosols, small plumes of airborne particles much like a tiny hurricane. There are blood and body fluids on the instruments that are passed back and forth. Blood flows down the surgical drapings.

And all that blood surrounding me is deadly if my patient happens to be positive for AIDS. Am I allowed to know that? No.

That is the medium in which all surgeons function. To a less dramatic extent, that is the hazardous environment in which 6.5 millions of health care workers toil.

Add to that grim number legions of firefighters, rescue workers, police officers, ambulance crews and school nurses, and the statistics increase radically.

The nurses, residents and interns who assist me in the operating room have dreams, hopes, lives ahead of them, young children. As the November 13, 1989, *San Francisco Chronicle* described this battlefront environment in which I stand and try to talk some sense into ears that have been deafened by AIDSpeak: "—imagine wondering whether sometimes there might be something lethal in the blood rising like fog from the patient, a contagion that worms its way into human cells, *yours,* and waits, sometimes for years, to attack and then maybe to kill."

Imagine that a surgeon or dentist who has contracted the disease and doesn't know it yet, or who may know but will not tell for fear of losing patients, is doing surgery on you.

He cuts or pricks himself with a sharp instrument or needle during surgery, small accidents that happen every week, as every operating staff will tell you, and bleeds a small amount of blood into your wound.

He could kill you.

Impossible, you say. This cannot be. These scenarios don't happen in America. After all, we have governmental watchdogs whose duty is to show-and-tell? There are safeguards. Isn't that what hospital environments are for, to protect both patients and health care workers from danger?

It happened a few months ago.

A dentist, fortified with mask and gloves, gave AIDS to a young patient. Said a nonchalant CDC official when interviewed about the case on national network TV, "We've known for some time that this was going to happen. *The real question is: Should we do something about it?*"

That's AIDSpeak—sidestepping the issue with vagueness or glossing it over with unfounded confidence. The government bureaucrats have become experts at AIDSpeak.

This book is about AIDSpeak and its many manifestations:

AIDSpeak proclaims that even if the news is bad, it means nothing. "Don't worry."

Before I started working on this book I did not realize how deep in our culture AIDSpeak has managed to take root. It gets its energy from something that we never discuss, unless we do so righteously, resoundingly and patriotically. That something goes by many names, but as often as not, it is called "human rights" or "confidentiality."

AIDSpeak translates into death.

When I accept a patient, both of my hands are bound. As a doctor entrusted with this patient's care, I am allowed to test without permission for any disease known to man—except AIDS.

As a patient, you have the right to know about your surgeon's schooling, lawsuits, professional track record, specialization and, I suspect, credit rating as well—practically everything except the fact that your surgeon may carry the virus that kills.

That's crazy.

How did we become so nonchalant? The answer is simple. We aren't taught that vigilance is virtue. We're taught that nonchalance is *chic.*

I know that when the AIDS epidemic was first identified in the early 1980s, we in the medical profession reacted in a cavalier manner. We knew in a tangential sort of way that the virus was transmissible by blood. We knew because a patient who was unfortunate enough to have received a blood transfusion that was contaminated with the virus was turning positive.

By and by some timid questions grew.

I remember beginning to feel a vague unease about blood-borne infection from patient to doctor as early as 1983. I would go to the infectious disease experts in my hospital and ask them, "Might there be a problem? Isn't it somewhat risky what we are doing in the operating room? We are getting blood all over us."

They would shake their heads like Brahmans and assure me, "No, no—Lorraine. No way."

I looked at them. They looked at me.

Their function was to track contagious diseases. My function was to operate.

Almost apologetically, I would push on. "But I do get a lot of needlesticks, you see?"

They insisted, "No. No way."

You couldn't get it from patient blood that soaked through your gown to your belly.

You couldn't get it from an injury such as a needlestick.

No way did it transmit through intact human skin.

You couldn't catch it if you tried, unless, of course, you were promiscuous or unlucky enough to get a large injection of HIV-positive blood.

I countered, "But I don't think you realize just what it is we do in the operating room."

Infectious disease specialists are not surgeons. Many have never been in any operating room during any part of their medical training. Their function is consultancy. They may see patients in a clinic or office but they don't routinely take primary care of patients on a hospital ward. They come around, read the charts, talk to the patient, and leave a note of consultation. They rarely do hands-on work in a hospital. If blood is to be drawn, it certainly is not the infectious disease consultant who draws the blood; it is the technician, the intern or the resident.

Repeatedly, I would go back to them and say, "You know, this does seem dangerous to me."

And they would respond, "No. No. You need more than a needlestick."

It is true that infectious disease doctors in some hospitals are heavily involved in treating AIDS patients, but that does not mean they are drawing blood or getting contaminated with patients' body fluids. They aren't soldiers in the trenches, but, on the other hand, they are my colleagues who have specialized in something I have not.

I had known them for years. I trusted them. I had no reason not to trust them.

And what they said to me, I blithely passed on to my surgical colleagues and students.

Since I was in a leadership position as Chief of the Orthopedic Surgery Service at San Francisco General, I would often get calls from other orthopedic surgeons across the country, asking worriedly whether or not there was any danger in occupational transmission.

"No way," I told my colleagues. "The danger is practically zero."

Today my comments make me flinch. I wish that I had spoken up much earlier. Now I realize it was foolishly trusting of me to assume that the infectious disease specialists were trained to do their job and willing to do it conscientiously: to watch out for my safety, my nurses' safety, my students' safety and my patients' safety, and even more importantly, the public's safety. I didn't read the infectious disease specialty journals. I had enough to do to keep up with the literature in my own specialty. In the beginning, I never gave AIDS that much thought. I had my turf and they had theirs and I would go back to the trenches.

All the while, the virus dug in among patients.

Meanwhile, the numbers of calls from other surgeon colleagues did not decrease.

Since it is estimated that some 20 to 40 percent of San Francisco's male population is homosexual, a fairly well-defined and self-contained community where the disease first struck with virulence, more and more orthopedic surgeons around the country would call on me for advice if they had an AIDS patient on whom they had to operate.

My colleagues would insist, "Lorraine, what are you doing for protection?"

I would tell them that I had properly consulted with the appropriate specialists and they had confirmed for me that there was no danger at all, although all the time we were practically swimming in the blood. They assured me, repeatedly, "No way."

"There is no way," I said. "There are four ways you can get the disease: from risky sexual intercourse, from contaminated needles, from blood transfusions, and by having it passed on from mother to child."

That's AIDSpeak.

I spoke it and I didn't even realize it. It had been filtered into me by repetition.

About that time, some vague, disturbing rumors started. We heard about a couple of nurses in some other hospital who claimed they had contracted the virus from accidental needlesticks.

The hospital grapevine, at that point, started to hum, and what it hummed was AIDSpeak.

If you really checked those nurses' private habits, it was said, you would discover that it was their "lifestyle," surely, and not one tiny needlestick. We could not in good conscience, we told each other, AIDSpeak-style, incriminate the needlestick.

That just wasn't the way that the HIV virus could be transmitted. It was almost immoral to think that it could be transmitted that way and crude in the extreme to say so. Enlightened professionals "knew" that the virus in question did not, could not, and would not transmit in the workplace.

Shortly thereafter, the Centers for Disease Control published a provocative case report on a nurse who apparently had managed, after all, to infect herself with a single needlestick.

This report didn't cause any stir. At my hospital, at least, this first official case report was downplayed.

Our betters told us with raised eyebrows, "How do you know what that nurse *really* did? How do you know that she didn't lie? It could have been a bisexual boyfriend. It could have been from shooting up."

There were a lot of clucking tongues that clucked of careless, unprotected sex and drugs. There was no Red Alert. There were no widely disseminated instructions that told us at that time that we must be careful.

The CDC did publish some guidelines in an infectious disease journal that surgeons rarely read. The rest was nonchalance that turned into grim history.

About that time, I hired a young orthopedic trauma fellow. He was going to get married and his bride-to-be was having serious reservations about moving from Tennessee to San Francisco.

They had seen some alarming footage on a television show. He called me for some reassurance and I gave him just that. I told him there was nothing to that information.

"There are many other risks in this hospital," I said, a well-respected medical authority to whom this novice looked up to for guidance, "but AIDS in the operating room is not one of them."

Of course, I was totally wrong.

In July of 1987, Dr. Julie Gerberding at San Francisco General Hospital published her article in the *Journal of Infectious Diseases*[1] showing that approximately 60 health care workers at San Francisco General Hospital, who had been stuck with HIV-positive blood, and 55 who had received splashes with HIV-positive blood had now been tested.

Not one of them, the research documented, had since contracted the disease.

Relief.

Then came the shock. On October 2, 1987, at a Chiefs of Service meeting at my hospital, we were informed by the infectious disease staff that a woman nurse in our hospital, apparently one of the subjects in the above-named research sample who had previously tested negative, had now turned positive—*infected from a single needlestick.*

I sat there, stunned.

My entire life passed before me. I thought to myself: "How am I going to escape getting this disease?" In the past six, seven years, I had been stuck a hundred times—and more. If I had gotten stuck with a contaminated needle, I could be dead.

I told myself at that point, "Either the infectious disease doctors did not know *and should have* or they *did* know, and they weren't telling us."

I told myself, "These are the same people who told me not so long ago that you couldn't get AIDS from a blood transfusion, and they turned out to be wrong.

"These people told me that seroconversion meant that you were positive but had 'only' a ten percent chance of getting full-blown AIDS, and that turned out to be false.

"They told me women couldn't get it heterosexually, yet women can, and do.

"These people told me only yesterday that children couldn't get it, and now we have infections in the womb.

"They tell me now that, while a needlestick can kill, *I still can't get it by coming in skin contact with urine, feces, semen, perspiration, tears or saliva?*"

I drew a common-sense conclusion. These folks were wrong before. It stood to reason they could be wrong again.

"How many times," I said to myself, "do I need to find out that so-called 'experts' have their information wrong before I start looking into this matter myself?"

This Chiefs of Service meeting was a small group meeting of about twelve or fifteen people. Most were not surgeons. Not one of them was swimming in blood as I was.

I stood up because I wanted maximum attention and I said, "This information changes everything. I was told all along that this could not happen. Now I think it is important to ask that my patients be tested, voluntarily, of course, and with informed consent."

Everybody at the table thought that was a sensible idea.

They all agreed that it was certainly within the law. It was within the rules and regulations of the hospital.

We had a special consent form that we routinely used when we asked a patient to sign up for a test. I confirmed that I wanted to start doing that. I said more, "I want to be tested as well. My residents want to be tested."

Folk wisdom has it that it is useless for the sheep to pass resolutions in favor of vegetarianism while the wolf remains of a different opinion.

So it was true for us, the surgeons and the residents who wanted to be tested. We came to realize that blood tests for AIDS, even for health care professionals assumed to be negative, were not exactly a popular notion. There was a very simple reason: Our university dreaded offending special interest groups. After all, we lived and worked in San Francisco. The city had its share of homosexual politicians with their huge gay constituencies. They didn't want us to touch their Pandora's box. My request was stonewalled for two weeks. I was very nervous. I'd had enormous exposure. In the end, we drew each other's blood.

A hospital administrator collected the specimens but then forgot to put them in refrigeration. Apparently, this was just negligence and oversight, but just the same, our blood grew moldy. No one cared; this did not allay our fears.

Blood had to be drawn all over again, and once again we waited.

Seven weeks after the meeting that gave us the bad news, with all of us sweating it out, the results finally came back: not one of us carried the virus.

"That meeting," said the *San Francisco Chronicle* in the article entitled, *The Doctor Who's Afraid of Blood,* by Jerry Carroll.

marked the beginning of Day's emergence from the obscurity of a physician and medical professor respected in her field, but not much known beyond, and her entry into the vortex of bitter controversy and dispute.

Day, now 52, came to be considered by many as a closet homophobe who lent a spurious medical authority to the pronouncements of knuckle-dragging conservatives hoping to herd gays with AIDS into internment camps with towers and razor wire.

I don't know about that. I never said that. I never thought that. I never even dream that crassly. I do believe in drastic measures, and so, I hope, will you when I have had my say in this small illuminating volume.

I speak from a scientific, medical perspective when I contend that we have no choice but to surround and nullify the virus while we can. We must. We have no choice at all.

If our philosophy asks us not to sacrifice that hallowed AIDSpeak tool, "confidentiality," while we stand by and watch people die by the hundreds of thousands, then we'd better scrutinize our premises.

The virus has no philosophy. The virus is neutral. The virus will move on, regardless of our dearly cherished attitudes regarding human rights and such. This is a war not of us against ourselves, contaminated by our "prejudices."

It's us against the virus.

I started asking every patient on the ward to be tested. Most patients willingly agreed.

But there was one young man, clearly high-risk, clearly homosexual, who set his jaw, glared at me and said, "You are my doctor. You have to take care of me. And you aren't testin' me for nothin'!"

I told him, "You have an ankle fracture that is in excellent alignment. You are in a long leg cast. That is the way you will be treated unless your ankle fracture loses alignment. Then we will have to operate on you."

It is acceptable and, in fact, conservative practice in all hospitals for ankle fractures that are in good alignment to be treated with a long-leg cast and without surgery.

It is also true that we at San Francisco General often

operate on ankle fractures in patients who come in from the streets and who might be unreliable with follow-up.

I made sure that this young patient understood that follow-up was critical. Indeed he did because he came back regularly. I saw his X-rays every time he came back and he healed without any problems.

But somehow, AIDSpeak got to him. He came to a peculiar conclusion.

I can only speculate on whether he came to his conclusion by himself or others helped him reach it. He went directly to a newsreporter and told a major San Francisco paper I had withheld a necessary operation from him because he refused to be tested for AIDS.

I was widely criticized for having "changed" my treatment on an AIDS patient. A newspaper article several days later headlined the controversy "Uproar Over San Francisco Doctor's Testing Policy," and my colleagues, who saw no problem whatsoever in voluntary testing as discussed in our initial meeting, now all hid under the table.

Various colleagues insisted, "We don't know what she is doing. She's making her own policy. We don't agree with it. She didn't check with anyone."

I said as calmly as I could to anyone who listened that my testing policy was voluntary testing with signed consent.

It made no difference.

I kept on saying: "Both means of treatment are acceptable. The outcome is the same."

My motives were suspect. My principles were questioned.

I pointed out to friend and foe alike, "There are no problems with this patient. Please note there are no problems."

The word was out. And AIDSpeak did the rest.

I became known to the world as "the first doctor who

refused to do surgery on a patient with AIDS."

I was a "homophobe."

Since I was working in San Francisco's only trauma hospital with a tremendous volume of patients, I did as many operations in one year as the average orthopedic surgeon might do in ten.

HIV-positive patients had started coming into our emergency rooms because they would get injured—like everyone else. They had been shot or stabbed, or they had fallen out of windows, and it was up to me to treat them. Like it or not, I knew I had better dig in and find my own facts.

This is what the *San Francisco Chronicle* wrote:

Her close search of the literature turned up bits and pieces of research that were known to the narrow circles of AIDS researchers but that she thought didn't get enough attention from health care workers.

Day began publicizing them herself. Among them:

* HIV infection in homosexual men at high risk may occur at least 35 months before antibodies can be detected, according to the June 1, 1989, *New England Journal of Medicine.*

* Tests of surgical gloves don't detect holes smaller than 10 microns in diameter, which would allow AIDS and other viruses to come into contact with the skin, according to the *Surgical Practice News* of August, 1988.

* The AIDS virus may actually be able to enter the body through skin contact, according to *The Lancet*[2] of Nov. 7, 1987.

There was more, a great deal more.

I now began to see how deep the AIDSpeak practice runs. The more I thought about this situation, the more I came to feel a real sense of betrayal from the medical establishment. I found all sorts of things that were not common knowledge but were well documented in the medical literature.

I found out, for example, that the virus is not "fragile"— far from it.

It can survive on a dry surface for as long as seven days.[3]

It survives freezing.[4]   It can transmit through saliva.[5] It can transmit through oral sex.[6]

It seems to have transmitted at least once through a bite that didn't break the skin.[7]

It has been found and judged infective on needles in amounts so minute that they look like "clean" needles.[8]

Some disinfectants formerly believed to denature the virus have proved not to be sufficiently strong.[9]

This information was very nicely documented. Much of the medical "reporting," however, was coming through in anecdotal forms of case histories or small studies.

But did we have, I asked myself, large and conclusive studies as recently as six, seven years ago that told us blood transfusions could transmit the virus?

Thousands of lives had been wasted because, early on, the "experts" told us in the most authoritative manner possible that blood transfusions did not pass on the virus.

That studies were not yet available on contamination via

perspiration, for example, or even airborne contamination did not preclude the possibility of danger. *The absence of studies might only indicate that no one suspected the danger.*

Nobody was looking—so far.

Meanwhile, I kept on asking that patients voluntarily be tested for the HIV virus. I argued that prevalence statistics were vital. I said I had the right to know. In fact, I had an obligation to know. How could we control transmission of a disease as dangerous as AIDS unless we knew who had the disease?

It seemed like ABC to me.

To many of my colleagues, and certainly to my administrators, it seemed that in their midst walked an anarchist.

I went ahead with voluntary testing, agreed upon by my patients. Overnight this, too, blossomed into a gargantuan political issue.

Nightline, a national television show, sent a crew to San Francisco General to interview members of the medical staff on the merits and demerits of voluntary testing for AIDS.

Nobody seemed to realize the petty politics involved.

The cameras were set up on the fifth floor. Everybody else was interviewed before I was called up. When finally the call came for me, I went up to the fifth floor, too, and waited for my turn. James Walker, who was interviewing for the introduction, came out into the hallway hurriedly and ushered me towards the elevator.

I asked, "Where are we going? All the cameras are in there."

He replied, "No, you and I are going outside."

I exclaimed, "But it's the middle of November! It's cold outside."

And that's when I was told: "When we asked to interview you, the hospital administration didn't grant us permission. They are not happy with what you are saying. They told us they would not allow you to speak in the building and, therefore, you will now be interviewed outside."

I thought: "Is this really happening? How can this be?"

Here I was. I thought I had freedom of speech. All I was asking for was voluntary testing which was totally within the rules. I could not say that on the air? They were not going to let me speak in the building where I instructed our country's future doctors that they must test before they diagnose?

Well, so it goes.

If you look at that *Nightline* interview, I am the only one whose hair is blowing in the wind.

There were other subtle and not-so-subtle pressures.

While I was in the middle of an operation, getting yet additional exposure to blood and body fluids, a University of California attorney, Joe Cowan, called me up about the article in the *San Francisco Chronicle* and requested to speak with me.

As a nurse held the telephone to my ear because I was still scrubbed, Joe did not bother asking, "Is there any truth at all to all those allegations?"

He didn't ask how the patient's treatment turned out.

He didn't want to know my side of it.

Instead, he told me curtly that if I were sued for anything the article contained, I would have no malpractice insurance coverage.

I must admit that I was very alarmed.

All the while, nobody bothered to check the simplest facts with me; that I had not withheld treatment; that there was no injury to anybody for which I could be sued; that I never had refused medical care to any HIV-positive patient; and, that all I wanted was simple, voluntary testing with a signed, informed consent.

I wanted to know what diseases my patients might have so that I could monitor treatment. I also wanted to protect myself my nurses and my residents.

All to no avail.

My chairman, Dr. William Murray at UC San Francisco, called shortly afterwards and talked to the person who was my orthopedic fellow at that time, Dr. David Contreras.

Bill said to David, "You tell her that she has no choice. She is an employee of the university. She's got to operate on these patients!"

Instead of giving me orders through David, Bill could have picked up the phone and asked me: "Do you usually operate on ankle fractures?" Had he but asked, I would have told him: "Yes, I usually do. That doesn't mean I have to operate on every ankle fracture." He just barked his orders to be passed on to me and then went out of town for the weekend, leaving Dr. Harry Skinner in charge of the department.

Dr. Harry Skinner is an orthopedic surgeon who does not do trauma orthopedics or general fracture work regularly.

Dr. Skinner also called and talked to my secretary at San Francisco General Hospital, demanding that I call him. The people at UC, explained Dr. Skinner, wanted to see the films on the media-seeking patient, "so we can back her up on her diagnosis and treatment."

I knew what I was doing—and I knew that what I was doing was correct.

I had vastly more experience in this particular injury than

any of my colleagues over at the University Hospital. I treat ankle fractures all the time.

I was angry.

Here I was, spurned publicly by the committee that had initially privately supported a very sensible request, chastised by my department for which I had worked some 15 years, at a trauma hospital where I had routinely put in 80 hours a week, year after year, working all night and working all day, working much longer hours than the people did at the University and they were telling me, "You show us what you do and we'll pass judgment on your work—"?

Dr. Skinner called my secretary: "Calm her down! Calm her down!"

"She is perfectly calm," my secretary said: "It sounds like you people over there are ruffled up a bit."

Dr. Skinner ordered: "You have her call me!"

"Why should I call him?" I thought, "He doesn't pass judgment on what I do. I don't take my orders from him."

The following Monday, Dr. Murray, my chairman, was back.

A routine staff meeting was scheduled for that day. Because I was working across town at the General, I didn't arrive until the meeting had started to break up.

As I was rushing down the hall, several people on the staff were still there. They said to me: "Well. Well. We need to talk to you about last week!"

I looked from face to face and settled on Bill Murray.

Dr. Murray said, "Why didn't you call Harry Skinner?"

I saw no merit, as they say, in saving up my indignation for a rainy day. I glared angrily at my department chairman.

I said: "Look, Bill. Somebody could have said to me, 'You have been a valued employee of ours for over 15 years. Your medical judgement has never been questioned. Tell us your side of what is going on so that we can support you.' You just barked orders at me, and left town."

From that day on, there were all sorts of whisperings about me. The rumors flew. I was looked at with side-long glances by people who would pass me in the hallway.

I did get a letter from the house staff, the residents and interns. It was written on San Francisco General stationery but unsigned.

> At breakfast this morning, a group was discussing your actions regarding AIDS patients. In this political environment, we do not care to have our Department Chiefs know it, but we support your chosen course of action and we feel that you are doing us all a service. We know that a large number of residents and interns as well as other hospital employees support your efforts and appreciate them.

Here was a group of doctors who wanted to express support for how I was trying to protect them, and could they do it freely?

No. Their jobs would have been in jeopardy.

AIDSpeak got in the way.

About that time, there was an article in the American Medical News, a publication that goes to every doctor in the country, stating that I had called for mandatory pre-operative testing of patients. It said that I thought that surgeons had the right to know.

I received hundreds of letters from the medical community and, specifically, the surgical community from all parts of the United States supporting my stand. I was deluged with speaking invitations from surgical associations throughout the country.

"There's nothing in the Hippocratic Oath that says I have to sacrifice my life needlessly for the patient," I told them, and they supported me. It was comforting to know that I was not alone.

Meanwhile, back in my operating room, I started dressing up.

I started wearing a plastic face shield. I started wearing triple gloves. I put on double shoe covers, knee-high boots, reinforced disposable gowns, additional sleeve covers.

Then came the space suit.

Nothing I had done so far would cause me so much grief and notoriety on one hand, and so much subsequent support on the other.

By way of background, an article in 1988 in the *Journal of the American Medical Association*[10] led me to question whether the surgical face mask and plastic face shield were protection enough. The article was about the use of a laser on venereal warts. It warned that intact human papilloma virus DNA, the cause of venereal warts, was found in the aerosol smoke plume created by laser procedures used to remove the warts, and the virus was small enough to pass through a surgeon's mask.

I asked myself at that point: "What if the AIDS virus also can become airborne with the use of power saws and drills on blood-covered bone?"

The space suit itself was not really news. It was developed more than 15 years ago in Manchester, England, by Sir John Charnley, the orthopedic surgeon who developed the first total hip replacement. For over a decade, many orthopedic surgeons had worn them regularly while performing joint replacements to protect the patient from contamination from the surgeon's hair, skin and breath. It already contained mechanisms to filter the surgeon's breath as the air circulated back into the room. I simply asked for an additional filter for the air coming in from the bloody aerosols in the room—air that I was breathing in.

Now we had drama because we had visuals in a reverse situation—an orthopedic surgeon *protecting not just the patient from the doctor but herself from the patient!*

Nothing so propelled me right into the public eye as wearing that protective spacesuit. It catapulted my campaign for greater safety for the health care workers of America right onto *60 Minutes*.

My colleagues had this to say in the *San Francisco Chronicle*:

> "I can't say that the AIDS virus is not transmitted by an aerosol," says Dr. White (then president of the California Medical Association). "It's tough to prove a negative. But I don't know of any evidence that it is. But she's scaring the socks off people."

> "There would be a lot more physicians with AIDS if it could be transmitted as easily as Day fears," he said.

Her boss at San Francisco General, Dr. Merle Sande,

chief of staff, said Day "has fanned the hysterical parts of our personalities and has been destructive in that respect, but I respect her right to her views."

Just for the record: Dr. Sande was my colleague, not my "boss."

Dr. Mervyn Silverman, the former Director of Public Health for San Francisco, said if the disease could be spread through intact skin it would be far more prevalent. "Isn't it interesting that she is standing somewhat alone? One would think that if she were somewhat in the mainstream, there'd be support for her from some medical organization."

I had never planned to become a public spokesperson in this matter.

I genuinely thought, in the beginning, that I was working through hospital channels, in quiet meetings, obeying the rules.

At least at first, I was checking with everybody in the committee meeting even though it was perfectly legal to test for any illness on any patient needing to have treatment, as long as the patient agreed.

It saddens me to say, my colleagues hung me out to dry.

They could have said in public what each of them said in private, that a responsible and thorough surgeon has every right on earth to test with the patient's consent if testing helps the doctor make a more accurate diagnosis.

To omit a medical test for a deadly disease for political reasons is, at the very least, contributory negligence from the patient's point of view. Omitting such a test will put the health care staff treating an infected patient at added risk for a disease that has, so far, no vaccine, only token treatment and no cure.

I realized I was on my own. I had to do things in accord with my own nature and in accord with what my training had taught me.

A friend of mine said recently, "What you are saying is unpopular. It's not the party line. You will be viciously attacked. It is not going to be pretty. If you could wave a magic wand, what would it be?"

Ah, yes. If only there were choices. If only there were options.

I said, "I'd much prefer to be a stand-up comic. I'd love to tell some jokes! It's not pleasant to give people bad news."

There it is. Fate played a trick on me.

I am an orthopedic trauma surgeon, fixing broken spines, legs, arms, and other broken bones, teaching students, writing articles for medical journals, studying the literature to keep informed, giving lectures at conventions, giving testimony pertinent to my profession and conviction, fighting AIDSpeak everywhere, but it would be much more enjoyable to make a lot of people laugh!

What I see is not a laughing matter. The pit we dug ourselves is deepening and what will tumble in, the mind refuses to believe.

2

AIDSpeak in Action

The poster was pink. It was tacked to a bulletin board. I saw it in passing but didn't pay any attention to it.

I was busy with my duties when one of my friends, who happens to be a homosexual male, brought me the flyer and said: "Lorraine, did you see this on the wall?"

"Yes."

"Do you know where that is?"

"No."

"You can't let this happen! This is bad blood!"

"What do you mean?", I asked.

"This is Collingwood," answered my friend, "off of 18th Street, behind CALA Foods. That's where gay men take each other in the bushes at night. That's where a lot of sex takes place. And that's where they're having this blood drive. This blood drive is going to be in the heart of the Castro, Lorraine."

I took the poster, found a phone and called the phone number given for "Bob." I listened to a recording of an obviously gay male asking other men to come and bring their partners. He spoke of the "great fun" they were going to have.

He said that there would be a party—to come, bring a friend and give blood.

It was a message clearly directed at gay men. There was no doubt about that.

It is important to understand that the AIDS test used on blood bank blood is a test for the antibody to AIDS. It usually takes at least three months and sometimes as long as three years for an infected person to develop antibodies. So blood that is really positive can test negative. There is no commercially available test for the AIDS virus itself.

The Castro district in San Francisco has the highest per capita rate of AIDS infected individuals in the nation. How could any blood bank, in good conscience, schedule a blood drive in this area. Life in the Castro goes something like this.

Castro Street on Friday night looks like the furthest spot from human misery.

Young men stroll arm in arm to a noisy backdrop of music and traffic. There is laughter and the kind of familiar exchanges one expects to hear on Main Street of a small town. The crowd ebbs and flows through the neighborhood, passing the Cock A Doodle Doo restaurant, Does Your Mother Know card shop and Moby Dick bar.

The laughter is a facade that can't mask stark reminders that this neighborhood—home to San Francisco's gay community—is the epicenter of the nation's AIDS epidemic.

Ten years after AIDS appeared, there is no escaping the dozens of posters announcing AIDS fundraising events. Conversations about medical treatments, funerals and lost lovers can be overheard in bars and restaurants.

ARM IN ARM'S THIRD QUARTERLY

AIDS BLOOD DRIVE

Saturday, July 30th*

EUREKA VALLEY REC CENTER
Collingwood off 18th Street (behind Cala Foods)

10 AM—4 PM

Call for pre-registration and questions
863-9730 (Penni)   552-9574 (Bob)

Bring ID!   Bring a Friend!
Gifts and Prizes!

Sponsors: Java Road Trading Co.
Metro Video
Rossi's Meats

*changed from July 23rd so as not to conflict with AIDS Walk

Condoms and brochures promoting safe sex practices are easier to find here than candy bars.

Life has gone on in the Castro, but it is changed forever.

Researchers believe that half the gay men here— about 40,000 to 60,000 people—are virus carriers. They give the city the highest AIDS rate in the nation.

In the decade since AIDS was discovered, 8,459 residents of San Francisco have developed the disease; 5,580 have died. Almost 95 percent have been gay or bisexual men.

While there is no apparent preoccupation with the rising toll, virtually no one in the gay community has escaped the effects of the disease.

"All of my old friends have died," said Cleve Jones, a prominent gay leader. "I have no one left in my life, other than my family, who knew me before the epidemic."

. . . those who are now becoming sick were probably infected in the early 1980s, experts agree. The disease can incubate up to 10 years before symptoms appear.

Gannett News Service,
as reported on page 1 in the *Stockton Record*
June 17, 1990

I wrote a letter on July 21, 1988, to Herbert Perkins, M.D., executive director of the Irwin Memorial Blood Bank in San Francisco, a non-profit enterprise at that time still run by the San Francisco Medical Society. I voiced my objection as follows:

The attached notice is now posted on our bulletin boards at San Francisco General Hospital. I called the phone number listed and got a recording explaining that this indeed is a blood drive.

For the past twenty years the park adjacent to the Recreation Center has been a popular "cruising place" for individuals who live in the Castro area.

With the latent period for production of HIV antibodies now extended to 3 years, and thus an increased possibility for truly positive blood to test negative and be included in the donor blood supply, how prudent is it for the blood bank to participate in a blood drive in this area?

I received no response.

I sent copies to the director of our blood bank at San Francisco General Hospital, the Administrator of our hospital, Phil Sowa, the Chief of Staff, Dr. John Luce, the Chief of Medicine, Dr. Merle Sande and the Chief of Surgery, Dr. Frank Lewis.

I received no response.

Four or five days before the scheduled blood drive—and still waiting for an answer to my letter, I called the blood bank. I learned that Dr. Perkins was out of town. I talked to a man named Dr. Busch who was second-in-command. I asked Dr. Busch if Dr. Perkins had received my letter, and Dr. Busch responded, "Yes."

"I received no answer," I indicated.

"Well," said Dr. Busch, "Dr. Perkins is out of town."

I said, "Oh, he is? Well, do *you* think that it is prudent to go to the Castro to get blood?"

Dr. Busch said, "No, I don't."

"Well, then" I asked, *"Why* are you doing it?"

"There's no way," explained Dr. Busch, "that we can

cancel this blood drive. The gays would have a fit. We would get all sorts of bad publicity. We just can't do it! We just can't cancel it."

I explained to this man, "I don't want to give my patients this blood. Even my gay male patients don't want this blood. This is bad blood and you know it is bad blood."

Dr. Busch said again, "Well, we cannot cancel it. There would be too much bad publicity."

"In that case," I told Dr. Busch, "I think the people of San Francisco have the right to know where you are getting their blood."

"Well, if you are going to sensationalize it—" said Dr. Busch, and I countered, "I am not going to sensationalize it. I just think the people of San Francisco have the right to know where you are getting their blood."

Hesitantly Dr. Busch replied, "Well, give me a couple of hours, then—" and I went back to my work.

Dr. Busch never called me back. I did receive a call three or four hours later from Irwin Memorial's director of operations, Vince Yalon, who uttered something to the effect that I had caused them a great deal of trouble.

I exclaimed, "Pardon me?"

"You interfered in our blood drive," Mr. Yalon informed me.

I explained to Mr. Yalon: "I did not schedule this blood drive. You scheduled the blood drive. If you think it's safe, then you go ahead and I will just let the San Francisco public know. They can judge for themselves whether they think it's safe blood or not."

"Well, no," said Mr. Yalon. "No, no. We are going to cancel the drive."

I said, "Fine. Then that's the end of it!" and once more went back to my work.

It is true that I threatened to go to the media but, in fact, I never did. I considered the subject closed, glad that the blood bank had finally acted responsibly, and I saw no need to notify the citizens of San Francisco. It was the gay community that went to the media, and the media descended on me.

Television cameras suddenly showed up on my doorstep. Reporters half my age and with no medical background whatsoever wanted to know in so many words, "Who do you think you are when you know we have responsible people at the blood bank saying that the blood drive in the Castro is OK?"

I tried to shed enlightenment about the dangers of the situation, and the reporters asked, in turn, "Well, do you think that *anybody else* agrees with you on this?"

I pointed out to them: "They canceled the blood drive— didn't they?"

And I was told to my amazement, "No, they did not. They are sending vans down to the Castro. They are busing the donors out of the Castro to blood bank headquarters at Irwin Memorial to donate their blood there."

The blood drive was scheduled for July 30, 1988. Two days earlier, two major television stations featured the exploding controversy on prime time evening news. Within days if not hours the story was covered in the San Francisco media. The politicians rallied. The gay press was vociferous. The letters to the editor kept sizzling. The medical community was taking a leisurely cruise to the moon.

Out of all of this commotion emerged several telling

slants. They illustrate how, once again, a simple medical precaution regarding AIDS can become a gigantic political summit for AIDSpeak, at least in San Francisco.

First, it was said, over and over, that the blood drive was, in fact, a lesbian drive and lesbian blood was very safe—it was safer than general blood. The latter happens to be true—but nowhere did it say on the poster and nowhere was it stipulated that only lesbians were recruited and would donate at that location.

In truth, it was an open blood drive in the Castro. The Irwin Memorial blood bank admitted it. I know, because I asked.

Second, it was repeated everywhere that the blood donated was earmarked for the AIDS-infected gay community, the PWAs (People With AIDS). In fact, it was blood collected for general inventory that could have gone to Iowa, since blood banks have a flourishing exchange system within all states and even across borders. To this day, the U.S buys some blood from Mexico.

And, finally, it was shrieked in language I have never seen applied to any medical professional, particularly one who simply asked for a common-sense precaution regarding a communicable and 100 percent lethal disease. Lorraine Day, M.D., Chief Orthopedic Surgeon of San Francisco General Hospital was labeled as media-hungry, homophobic, medically incompetent and woefully deficient, ethically and morally.

That summer was no fun. I learned to my dismay that one can make an easier living as a soothsayer than as a truthsayer. The attacks on my personal motives and professional integrity proved relentless.

Rather than paraphrase the sequence of events and reconstruct the chronology and nature of the controversy, I will simply let some letters, articles and news releases give an echo of the escalating shrillness of AIDSpeak.

San Francisco's Mayor Art Agnos was one of the first to speak out against me.

In a letter addressed to Dr. Herbert Perkins, head of the Irwin Memorial Blood Bank and reproduced in the *Bay Area Reporter,* the city's major gay newspaper, Mayor Agnos spoke ringingly of his conviction that the Castro blood drive was democracy in action, worthy of the judicious stance on AIDS for which his fair city was known:

> I would like you to know that I fully support your decision that Irwin Memorial Blood Bank should conduct blood drives in all areas of the city, including in the Castro, using the full array of safeguards which have been developed.

> When I served in the California State Assembly, I was impressed with your professionalism and dedication to those in need of safe blood transfusions. I welcomed and appreciated your assistance and support for my legislation, which put into place the first requirements for testing blood for HIV antibodies. As you know, we drafted that legislation to provide state-of-the-art public health guidelines to protect all the public.

> I have discussed the concerns raised about the current blood drives in the Castro with Dr. Don Francis, who is serving as a special consultant to me on AIDS. He concurs that the public health is well protected with the safeguards that have been in place.

> In view of the objections raised, it is important to

note that the first line of public health defense has been the extremely strong level of cooperation from the lesbian and gay community that no one possibly infected should donate blood.

In addition to this very successful self-deferral program, the blood supply is further safeguarded by an intensive interview at the time of donation, when an option to discreetly withdraw or earmark a donation for research rather than human use is provided.

A battery of tests also is applied to blood donations, including tests with the most sensitive assay test available for HIV and additional tests for markers to the hepatitis B virus, which often appears in those with HIV infections.

As I will show, these tests are not completely reliable. There exists what is known as the "negative window"—more fully explained in subsequent chapters. *The negative window is the time span between infection that has occurred and infection that can be detected. It can be as long as three-and-a-half years.*

The public, reading the mayor's reply, would not have known that, even with the best of testing programs, HIV could easily have found its way into the general blood supply.

The letter went on to say:

The level of volunteerism from the lesbian and gay community to combat the HIV epidemic has saved lives in our city. Indeed, they have carried much of the burden for educating the rest of the city about risks and safeguards.

In view of that record, I am dismayed by proposals that imply that groups which have performed such a public service are unreliable in serving the larger public health needs.

In the past, Irwin Memorial Blood Bank has performed its important role in our community with dignity and professionalism. I know you will want to continue to place your focus on genuine public health rather than a political or public relations response to the epidemic.

If there is any assistance which you believe that I, as mayor, might provide to your organization in meeting its public health goal, please call on me.

That's AIDSpeak at its finest.

It was seconded in spirit, word and letter by Mervyn Silverman, former Director of Public Health of San Francisco, Don Francis, M.D., a Centers for Disease Control AIDS consultant to the mayor, David Werdegar, M.D., San Francisco Director of Public Health and many others in the highest echelons of our nation's health care system, along with scores of my medical colleagues.

Gay people vented their feelings of outrage in their letters to the editor:

I am shocked that the intervention of one city employee, Ms. Lorraine Day of San Francisco General, could subvert a Castro area blood drive.

In the past Ms. Day has insisted all surgery patients at S.F. General be tested for HIV. Her rationalization was that she was free to withhold or dispense medical care on the basis of her personal preferences and that there was a danger to her by blood during surgery.

As to her choice of choosing patients, such an act is not only a violation of her medical oath of ethics, it certainly must be a violation of the policies of a publicly funded hospital.

If she finds herself unable to prevent infection by blood-born (sic) diseases, she had best find another occupation. Clearly her professional competence as a surgeon is highly suspect if this is the case.

The letter above was titled: "A Violation of Ethics." On the same page was another letter, urging me creatively: "Physician Day, Heal Thyself."

It ran as follows:

I see the AIDS-phobic Dr. Lorraine Day, an orthopedic surgeon at San Francisco General Hospital, strikes again! At her urging, two very important blood drives benefiting PWAs were cancelled because she believes Castro blood to be tainted. Did she take time to investigate that the donor base of these drives do not include high-risk individuals, but instead are predominantly lesbian, a population with the lowest incidence of HIV infection? Is she qualified to dictate blood donor policy by her position? She has also been making the rounds on the talk show circuit advocating mandatory testing for hospital patients. Dr. Day dismisses counter arguments by pompously displaying her credentials as a physician when her opponents lack M.D. at the end of their signature. Yes, Dr. Day has her First Amendment right to voice her opinion, but where was a more enlightened response? Why is San Francisco General Hospital silent?

Looking at the Hippocratic Oath one can read "First, do no harm." The ill-considered involvement of Dr. Day in matters unrelated to her specialty has done harm to the many PWAs who would have benefited from the lesbian community's outstanding efforts.

Her opinions are the thing tainted—poisoned by AIDS-phobia. Physician, heal thyself!

A few days after the blood drive, I wrote to KPIX, a San Francisco television station that had been guilty of biased reporting. That letter, dated August 2, 1988, is partially reproduced here:

I was quite disappointed in your coverage of the Castro district blood drive on Thursday, July 28. It seemed to be very one-sided, particularly by not mentioning the following points:

Nowhere on the poster was there any mention that this was a Lesbian blood drive.

The blood obtained in the blood drive goes into the general blood supply—it does not go specifically to AIDS patients.

On the poster is "Bob's" phone number. I called it and got a recording that was obviously directed to gay males.

The blood drive was being held at the exact spot (18th and Collingwood, behind Cala Foods) where gay males cruise at night and take sexual partners (multiple, if one wishes) into the bushes. If you doubt my word I suggest you go there some evening and see for yourself.

My only goal is to have as pure a blood supply as possible for all the citizens of San Francisco—including you, your family and all of my patients, many of whom are gay.

I am only trying to persuade the medical community, the media and the general public to handle this epidemic with medically sound principles, rather than letting special interest political groups take over.

Unfortunately, I have found that most people are so afraid of being called a bigot that they have lost their common sense.

I still had not heard from Dr. Herbert Perkins, executive director of the Irwin Memorial Blood Bank. I asked the director of San Francisco General's blood bank, Dr. Pearl Toy, what she knew about official policy regarding soliciting blood in the Castro. She assured me that Irwin Memorial was cognizant of the dangers of location and careful regarding where blood was being drawn. She said that she believed it was the policy of Irwin Memorial *not* to conduct a blood drive in the Castro.

I wrote another letter to Dr. Herbert Perkins:

Because you were out of town last week and unavailable, I asked Dr. Pearl Toy if it was usual procedure for Irwin Memorial to go to high risk areas for blood drives.

If I understand her correctly, she is under the impression that the official policy of Irwin Memorial is not to go to areas such as the Castro or the Tenderloin for blood drives.

However, the gay man speaking on Channel 4 on Friday's 5 p.m. news stated that Irwin Memorial has been going to the Castro for blood regularly for the past 4 years.

I have the following questions:

What is your policy on blood drives in the Castro or in the Tenderloin? What is your policy on busing people from the Castro or the Tenderloin to Irwin Memorial to donate blood?

Isn't it true that the blood from Saturday's drive in the Castro goes to the general blood supply and not just to AIDS patients?

Where on the poster does it mention that this is a lesbian blood drive? I phoned "Bob" and heard a recording that was obviously directed towards gay males.

If it is indeed your policy to have blood drives in the Castro, why did you spend money to bus the blood donors to Irwin Memorial? Why not stand firm that the Castro is a good place to get blood?

(The Tenderloin is the San Fancisco area most highly populated with drug addicts.)

I kept waiting for a response.

The widening controversy was depicted in a homosexual local newspaper.

"Bring the Blood Drive Back to the Castro," urged another gay newspaper, the *San Francisco Sentinel*, the next day:

The decision by Irwin Memorial Blood Bank last week to transfer the Arm in Arm donor drive out of the Castro was a shameful capitulation to the politics of fear over reason. It is a decision that demands to be repudiated by all segments of the city's medical and governmental leadership.

Three times this year, Arm in Arm has successfully recruited blood donations from women, primarily lesbians, as part of Irwin Memorial's designated donor drive. The beneficiaries of the drive are AIDS patients who need blood transfusions.

Not true. Until this controversy started and exploded, there was no effort whatsoever to recruit blood only from the lesbian pool, as I will show, nor was there any mechanism locked in place that set aside the Castro blood for persons infected with AIDS.

It was simply assumed this was so, and repeated over and over. The article continued:

The success of the drive and the safety of the blood collected are amply demonstrated by Irwin Memorial's decision to return repeatedly to the Eureka Valley Recreational Center to conduct additional drives.

This year, however, the drive fell victim to the inflammatory rhetoric of Dr. Lorraine Day, an orthopedic surgeon at San Francisco General Hospital, who threatened a media war denouncing the drive for occurring in a "high-risk community." Despite a preponderance of evidence to the contrary, Day tried to fan the flames of fear and bigotry by attesting that the drive would in some way endanger the safety of the blood supply.

Rather than refute Day's baseless assertions, Irwin Memorial responded with an awkward arrangement of shuttling donors attracted to the site in the Castro to its headquarters on Masonic Avenue. It was a pointless exercise which had no beneficial effect on the safety of the blood collected in this manner. All it achieved was a sharp reduction in the volume of donations, thereby penalizing the PWAs who would have been the ultimate recipients.

Irwin Memorial's decision to move the drive also sent a dangerously wrongheaded message to the public— both in San Francisco and the country—that perhaps Day's description that neighborhoods can put people at risk of AIDS has some validity.

Neighborhoods *can* put people at risk.
The Tenderloin in San Francisco would be a prime example. It is an area infested with drug pushers and prostitutes. No blood bank should go there. No blood bank should hold drives in areas where there might be a high concentration of Haitians or hemophiliacs.

Why should the Castro with its overwhelmingly gay population be different? And why was there a sudden "decrease" in the number of donors? Could it be that high risk males perceived themselves now under scrutiny?

But to continue:

Irwin Memorial inadvertently has given Day a validity she could have never hoped to achieve otherwise.

As of today, the decision has been made by Irwin Memorial to transfer the Milk Club Drive out of the Castro. But the *Sentinel* has learned that decision is under review and may be reversed.

There is still time for Irwin Memorial and the City to redeem itself by rejecting Lorraine Day's appeal to ignorance. The blood bank and the city should endorse the Milk Club drive in the Castro.

(Harvey Milk was a gay politician.)

While I was pondering this onslaught of AIDSpeak and trying to maintain a modicum of perspective in the wake of such irrational passion, another headline in the Bay Area Reporter, written by Allen White, caught my eye.

"Castro Blood Unsafe, Says Blood Bank: Irwin Admits Pressure from Day Forced Move to Masonic."

> The fourth annual *Women's Day Blood Drive* is being forced out of the Castro this weekend. The drive will be held Saturday from 10 a.m. to 4 p.m. at the Irwin Memorial Blood Bank at 270 Masonic at Turk. Shuttle buses will take people from the Castro to the Masonic location. . . .
>
> As the controversy has mounted, Irwin Blood Bank staff are now admitting that their blood supply is, in fact, not completely safe. Following meetings with Irwin Memorial executive director Dr. Herbert Perkins, Maurice Belote, president of the *Harvey Milk Lesbian/ Gay Democratic Club*, said, "Dr. Perkins has always been the first to say that the blood supply is inherently not safe. Any time you are dealing with the human blood, there is always great risk, and when a physician is faced with giving a person blood, that physician always considers the risks and the benefits."
>
> Irwin director of operations Vince Yalon said, "Even the slightest suggestion that the blood bank might be compromising the safety of community blood supplies is enough to warrant a change in perspective. In this case, it meant changing the location of the blood drive."

Sylvia Ramirez, an Irwin spokesperson, said, "To appease Dr. Lorraine Day and to try and work this thing out, we decided to move the site of the blood drive out. We didn't think it would make the blood safer, we just thought it would calm her down while we had a chance to get our act together and go back and talk and reason with her."

Throughout the entire controversy, nobody ever talked with me. None of my medical colleagues publicly supported my stand. They treated me as though I had done the unspeakable, the equivalent of having taken out a membership in, say, the Ku Klux Klan, although later, privately, virtually all of them agreed with me.

There was something almost surreal about that summer, as though people had conspired to turn all rules of safety upside down, insisting they were right side up. At fault was *my* perception. To say the least, it was bizarre, uncomfortable personally, and an assault on my integrity as a physician.

(Dr. Day) was listened to, says Ramirez, "because she is chief of orthopedic surgery at San Francisco General, and she uses the product we collect, and because we just couldn't ignore the suggestion that we might be compromising the blood supply. To have a physician with her credentials out there telling people that blood is unsafe and that we are collecting from unsafe donors in an area that is perceived as the highest HIV-positive district in the city, that is going to carry a lot of weight. What Dr. Day is saying is that we are holding it in an area where people could walk off the street, people who might be at risk for AIDS, it might be an invitation for people who are at high risk for AIDS to donate."

Ramirez justified the change in location, saying, "You know, sometimes we do things that have no scientific basis. We are responding to a person who has kind of an irrational fear. . . . Sometimes you have to do things that don't make a whole lot of scientific sense."

Concerning the blood supply from Irwin, she added, "There is no 100% testing for AIDS or hepatitis or anything. We can say that we have tested it to the fullest of our ability. I don't think anyone knows the answer to that question . . . . That is not to say that we will never find out. People who have been transfused don't get AIDS right away. It may take several years."

Indeed it does. In June of 1989, the *San Francisco Chronicle* reported the findings first documented in the *New England Journal of Medicine* on page 1458:

The AIDS virus may lurk undetected for as long as three years in the blood cells of some infected men, even though standard antibody tests indicate that the men are still uninfected. . . .

The Los Angeles researchers studied 133 of those men, all of whom continuously registered negative on the standard tests that detect antibodies to HIV, the human immunodeficiency virus.

In nearly one-quarter of the men, the virus was isolated, grown in laboratory cultures and clearly identified. . . .Four of the infected men who showed no antibodies to the virus had carried the organism in their bloodstreams for 11 to 17 months until standard antibody tests did show they were positive for infection, while the rest remained negative for as long as 35 months.

In the summer of 1988, a UPI release summarized at least some of these very frightening findings:

> As many as one in every 5,000 people who undergo major surgery may become infected with the AIDS virus from tainted blood that slips through the screening process, according to new research.
>
> In areas where AIDS is more common, the risk may be as high as one out of every 500 to 1,000 people who require large amounts of donated blood. . . .
>
> The risk stems from the fact that tests used to screen donated blood for HIV fail to pick up all infected blood because people do not produce antibodies to the deadly virus for at least several weeks after they have been infected.

Less than two weeks after my protest—and while my folder on unsafe blood grew thicker and thicker and thicker—Allen White of the *Bay Area Reporter* kept needling:

> Leaders Urge Donors: "Write Protest Letters to Irwin Blood Bank"
>
> Lesbian and gay leaders urged community members Tuesday to write letters of support for a return of blood drives to the Castro neighborhood. The appeal came as Irwin Memorial Blood Bank's board of directors planned a meeting for Aug. 11 to discuss an issue which was highlighted by recent demands from a San Francisco physician who wants to keep the blood drives out of the

predominantly gay and lesbian Castro.

Dr. Lorraine Day . . . recently had threatened a "media war" unless Irwin discontinued blood drives in the Castro. Day was successful in her campaign, which she took to several media outlets in the area. A result was that several local news organizations reported that "gays were giving blood in the Castro."

Since Day's demands started, Irwin relocated its blood drive to its own offices, 15 blocks from the Castro. But Lenore Chinn, coordinator of the AIDS/ARC Blood Fund for the *Harvey Milk Lesbian and Gay Democratic Club,* said the blood bank had opened the doors of communication in the dispute.

"Irwin Memorial is bending over backwards to help us," said Chinn. "Dr. (Herbert) Perkins recommends returning the blood drive to the Castro, but he also urges interested members of the community to write to the [blood bank's] board of directors."

Perkins confirmed Chinn's statement. "I would be delighted to present letters supporting the Milk Club's position to our board," Perkins said. "I am supportive of their position."

Indeed. For reasons that are still somewhat mysterious to me, given the extent of AIDS infection in the gay community, gay males are more-than-willing blood donors. And for years they have been courted by the blood banks. Why? The majority of homosexuals, because of their anal sex and multiple partners, are positive for antibodies to hepatitis B. The blood banks need those antibodies for one of the blood products they manufacture.

Furthermore, as far as a blood bank is concerned, a willing

donor is an inexpensive donor, since less money needs to be spent on recruiting.

> Lesbians and others who are in low risk groups for AIDS have held blood drives in the Castro for the last several years. That would all come to a stop as the blood bank reacts to charges that blood given in the Castro is tainted. Chinn reports that "better than 95 percent" of all Castro donors are lesbians.

A friend of mine recently gave blood at the Castro location. She and a male donor were the only two donors present. She knew about the controversy that erupted some three years ago. She pointed to some lesbian literature and inquired, "Is this a lesbian drive?"

"Oh, no," she was told. "We encourage both males and females to donate."

"It seems pretty empty here, doesn't it?" she asked.

A male attendant explained it to her: "You know how it is among us. Most people have busy schedules, *but those of us who know how important this drive is come early to donate. Many have been here already.*"

The article above continued:

> The Castro district, as a blood donation site, provides a comfortable, nonclinical, and supportive environment to our target population, which often prefers to have its activities and identity anonymous.
>
> They (blood bank authorities) noted that the drive is successful because it is viewed as being sensitive to the considerations of the prospective donors.

They also pointed out that the drive provides a blood fund for people with AIDS and ARC, to offset the financial burdens they face.

The Women's Day Blood Drive has been honored by groups and civic officials ranging from former Mayor Dianne Feinstein and the board of supervisors to the Roman Catholic Church. . . . Since 1985 the *Milk Club Women's Day Blood Drive* has issued over 500 credits to people with AIDS and ARC. . . .

Chinn said that if the Irwin blood bank bows to the pressure tactics of Day, "a frightening precedent may be set." Chinn noted that a domino effect would be set up, where people would start isolating the Castro, using the blood bank's directive as an example.

The scare tactics have become increasingly alarming because the blood bank has maintained that it has a screening process to isolate any unsafe blood. This includes blood infected with the AIDS virus. . . .

Maurice Belote, president of the *Milk Club,* said that the actions by the blood bank have created a concern by several elected officials. He said Mayor Art Agnos and (Supervisor) Harry Britt are aware of the problem. "They are very concerned, and their offices have been extremely cooperative," he said. For the last several days, he and other members of the club have been thrust into meetings with health officials where they have had to actually prove that the Castro is not an unsafe area for blood drives. "It is infuriating and a waste of time, but it has to be done," Belote said.

I reflected sadly on the knowledge that the blood banks had been wrong before. The blood banks told the nation's physicians many times prior to 1983 that the risk of blood-borne AIDS was negligible.

As it turned out, that was not true.

Once a blood test became available in 1985 that tested for the antibody to the virus, they said the same. The blood was safe. They said so even more vociferously.

As we now know, they are misleading the public again. The nation's blood bank inventory is *not* completely safe!

As a surgeon who had ordered blood transfusions on many occasions and would surely have to do so in the future, I was well aware of the shock and pain I had to inflict when that blood transfusion, meant to save a life, turned out to be AIDS-infected blood that would land the patient in the grave.

Those phone calls to my unsuspecting patients were sheer anguish for them and for me.

I remember having to work up my courage for days before I could pick up the phone and call a young mother to tell her, "You may have received contaminated blood. I would like you to come in for testing."

The *San Francisco Sentinel*, meanwhile, let me know that the Castro blood drive location was "pending."

Following last week's disruption of the *Arm in Arm* blood drive in the Castro, officials from Irwin Memorial Bank, *The Harvey Milk Club* and *Arm in Arm* met Tuesday in negotiations that both sides described as "very productive."

"We haven't made a permanent decision on whether the *Harvey Milk Club Women's Blood Drive* will take place in the Castro," said Dr. Herbert Perkins, executive director at Irwin Memorial. Perkins said that the decision would be made by Irwin's board of directors, and that he was trying to reach Washington Burns, the board president, to call an emergency meeting to resolve the matter. . . .

"I think we saw very much eye to eye," Perkins said of his meeting with blood drive administrators. "They are obviously being very careful. . . . The important point is not the area but who's trying to donate."

"It was a very productive meeting," said Bob Sokol, administrative director of *Arm in Arm.* "Perkins seemed very, very open to discussion. He seemed impressed by the fact that we were informed, intelligent, capable people, and that as much as lay people could, we were cognizant of the screening process, not some wackos off the street. I believe he is favorably disposed to getting us back [in the Castro.]

Sokol said the group discussed what they would do in the event that Dr. Day continued to "crucify us in the press." He said the group decided that "we would just as soon not validate her by mounting our own media blitz."

Lenore Chinn, coordinator of the upcoming *Women's Blood Drive,* said, "I don't think a decision will come in time to help us out." But Chinn added that Perkins seemed "extremely supportive" and that with enough letters of support to take back to his board, the decision could swing in favor of returning the drive to the Castro.

And so it did.

Less than four weeks after the re-shuffled drive, the *Bay Area Reporter* informed the gay community of San Francisco:

No Redlining Castro, Says Blood Bank

Irwin Memorial Blood Bank has reversed its recent policy of banning blood drives from the Castro area and will cooperate with two neighborhood blood drives in the future. Vince Yalon, director of operations for Irwin Memorial, confirmed that the blood bank will work with *Arm in Arm* and the *Harvey Milk Club Women's Day* blood drives. The next drive is scheduled for October.

"The blood drives are back in the Castro," said Maurice Belote, president of the *Harvey Milk Lesbian/ Gay Democratic Club.* . . .

A good five weeks after I had first voiced my concern about the Castro blood drive to the Irwin Memorial Blood Bank, I finally received a written reply from Irwin Memorial.

Dr. Herbert Perkins never called me on the phone. He never had the courtesy to talk to me about the controversy. He did meet with the homosexual groups, all of them lay people. But finally I did receive a letter.

It was dated August 29, 1988. I consider this letter unbelievable. Both it and the press release he included with the letter are quoted here in full:

Dear Dr. Day:

Forgive me for not replying to you sooner, but your first communication arrived just as I was leaving town to be a visiting professor at UC San Diego. I was not then familiar with the details of the mobile {blood drive} which concerned you, and I asked Vince Yalon, our Director of Operations, to check it out. Before I returned, you had already gone to the TV station.

As you are aware, Vince's response to your concern was to transfer the lesbian sponsored drives to the blood bank until I could return and confirm or alter our policies. On my return from San Diego I met with the organizers of the *Arm in Arm* and the *Harvey Milk* blood drives, and reassured myself that we were dealing with knowledgeable and responsible people who had no more desire to have units with HIV collected than would you or I. The decision to confirm previous policies was made hours before I left on the only two weeks of the year when it was possible for me to take a vacation. I regret that I did not make the time to respond to you before I left. I am enclosing a copy of a statement that I wrote just prior to leaving as a response to the inquiries which I knew were coming.

Your statements, as I am sure you are aware, resulted in innumerable letters and petitions addressed to me urging that the blood bank continue its previous policies of selected mobiles within the Castro district. Although I can attribute the large volume to the good organization of the gay and lesbian community, it is noteworthy that I received only a single letter of support of your position. In support of blood drives in the Castro by responsible groups were letters from the Mayor (citing Don Francis of the CDC to justify his support) and from a number of your colleagues at UCSF who are deeply involved in the fight against AIDS.

I accept the fact that your concerns have a sound basis; (italics added) I hope you will credit me with doing my very best to provide San Francisco with adequate amounts of blood that is as safe as possible. I have spent my entire career preaching that blood transfusions have serious side effects including risks of potentially lethal infections (and this was before AIDS). In terms of the risk of AIDS from blood collected in San Francisco, I do not believe it is now significantly higher than in other areas. For the last few years we have averaged three anti-HIV positives per 10,000 donors. That is not significantly different from the national average. More important, I think we can agree that the risk is primarily from those donors who are anti-HIV negative because they were recently infected. Thus, the primary determinant of risk should be the number of new infections in the area. Three different cohorts (groups) of gay men in San Francisco now show seroconversion rates of zero to 1% per year. (True. There are only a small number of *new* infections, because 75-80% of the homosexuals in these groups are *already* infected. *Ed.*) Another statistic which says that the risk here is low (but not zero) is the fact that we have only two recognized anti-HIV positive recipients since we began screening donors with anti-HIV in March 1985. And each of those two recipients has something in the medical history to raise a question about where the infection was acquired.

Now to respond to specific points in your letters: The *Bay Area Reporter* interview with Sylvia Ramirez is one of the worst examples of reporting I have seen—and I have been badly misquoted many times myself.

Sylvia (our Public Information officer) said that we had two cases of AIDS among recipients since testing for anti-HIV began (as I noted above).

Pearl Toy was obviously not correct when she said our policy did not permit any mobiles in the Castro area. You are correct that all blood goes into the same pool unless autologous or designated. I discussed with the organizers of the two blood drives the fact that their posters should be explicit about who may not donate. They agreed to cooperate.

I believe this answers all your questions. If not, please contact me.

Dr. Perkins also wrote to one of my colleagues at San Francisco General:

Plowing through the foot of correspondence I received about the Castro mobile, I found your FAX of July 29.

You were misinformed about our policy on going to the Castro. We did stop all mobiles to gay groups, but not those organized by lesbians.

I met with the organizers of the *Arm in Arm* and *Harvey Milk* drives. They have agreed to make their posters more explicit about who should not donate. I was impressed by the way they do advance screening on all donors (before our nurse does her screening). They know the people in the Castro and they are absolutely determined that no one at risk is going to slip through their net.

I am enclosing a copy of a news release I prepared in case we needed it.

The News Release was dated August 12, 1988, two weeks *after* the Castro blood drive.

> The Executive Committee of the Blood Bank Commission (the Irwin Board of Directors) reaffirmed today its continuing policy that blood drives will not be restricted as to the area in which they take place. The safety of the blood supply depends on the careful screening of the individuals who give blood, not the location where the blood drive is held. . . .

The Castro district in San Francisco continues to have the highest per capita of AIDS patients in the United States. (See illustration on following page.)

As of mid-1991, sad to say, the Castro blood drives are alive and well.

Illustration

Vincent Yalon, of the Irwin Memorial Blood Bank, in responding to a journalist's question on blood collection in the Castro, said "You can't make a decision based upon a zip code." How wrong he was.

Here is a "zip code" map published by the San Francisco Department of Public Health showing (outlined in black) the homosexual district, "the Castro", with the highest density of AIDS cases in the United States.

The 18th and Collingwood blood drive location is in the very center of this district.

SAN FRANCISCO EPIDEMIOLOGIC BULLETIN

CITY AND COUNTY OF SAN FRANCISCO • DEPARTMENT OF PUBLIC HEALTH • BUREAU OF COMMUNICABLE DISEASE CONTROL.

Vol. 1, No. 2   October 1985

AIDS Cases by Census Tract of Residence, First 1,000 Cases, San Francisco, 1981-1985

3

Bad Blood

The story has been "community spirit" for the good of the community—with no self-gain by those employed by the blood bank.

In actuality, no blood bank in the United States has ever gone bankrupt. They have all been profitable. They do not distribute their profits to the shareholders, (i.e. the public) but they certainly pay themselves handsome salaries with significant "perks."

The only concern the fresh blood provider has is this: "How can I get enough donors?" There is no trouble getting enough customers—i.e., every captive hospital in his territory is a customer. While self-limiting in the sense that there are a finite number of hospitals and a finite number of patients which may use a finite amount of blood, any business can operate profitably in a "known market"— particularly if monopolizing 100% of that market.

The limited source of donors, however, is a different

matter. The fresh blood sector uses one basic recruiting method which I refer to as the "guilt trip." There was a time when other motivations were used—that is, reduction in the hospital bill, free lunches, free dinners, grocery certificates, cash, etc. This is not so much done any more.

One inducement other than the "laying on of guilt" is still used today, although reduced somewhat by the currently strained economics of our society. Many unions include in their contracts with employers the stipulation that if a union member donates blood to the local blood provider, that employee gets half a day (or a full day) off of work with pay. This is particularly prevalent with government employees. Some inducement to donate may be pure pressure and competitiveness—that is, between groups, departments, etc.

Nevertheless, the basic message is the implication: "You are a terrible person if you don't help your fellow man who's going to die unless he gets your blood."

As expected, it is increasingly difficult for the fresh blood sector to recruit donors. As a result, blood banks do not want to reject donors for "minor" reasons—for example, mild infection, fast pulse, swollen lymph nodes, etc.

While every attempt is made to see that a donor qualifies within the limits set by law, no blood banks attempt to apply higher standards than those required by the law. Safer blood products at the expense of losing donors is resisted and justified on the grounds that a shortage of blood is more dangerous than the "long odds" of acquiring a blood-borne infection.

Donors are treated with kid gloves so as not to offend them. The blood bankers have resisted performing physical examinations which can be time-consuming or may reject and embarrass donors. The only driving force behind a blood bank's operation is "—we do not want to lose donors."

This economic factor is particularly important in understanding the basis of the lack of action of the fresh blood sector in 1983-85 and their almost criminally late recognition of the fact that AIDS can be transmitted by blood.

The passage above was written by an acquaintance of mine, a blood banker, one of the very few blood bank officials who spoke out fearlessly against the many lethal practices involved in the procurement, trafficking and sale of human blood.

I wish there had been more who had spoken out as he did. He clearly saw the not-so-hidden plunder that made for callous sacrifice of human lives for reasons many would call less than noble, and some might label criminal.

As one of the first physicians in the nation to voice suspicions publicly about contamination of our blood supply, I, too, became aware that there might be an operative factor that put public relations on a pedestal and human lives into the grave. It did not take me long to see that verified.

It's called the profit motive.

It happened from the start, and it's still happening. The Castro was just one example.

John Doe may not know, and if he were told, might not believe that this is so. The average American citizen, feeling chivalrous and selfless as he is having blood drawn from his vein in a blood bank drive replete with Red Cross, apple juice and doughnuts, believes that he is giving health and life to another human being.   Against that noble impulse, it is anathema to think of blood banks as corrupt.

Yet many of the actions of the nation's blood banks have been no less than sinister. They have been callously reactionary, irresponsible, calculated, negligent and profit-driven and, hence, malevolent.

To call them less than that does injustice to the many lives already lost and many who may still be lost.

How can that be?

Protocol stands in the way.   Special interest blackmail dictates policy.   Public image is believed to have a higher value than public safety.   The likes of Castro blood drives are palmed off as humanitarian enterprises when, in fact, they are concessions to gay politics.

Two examples illustrate my point. I summarize them here because they sketch the background of blood trafficking and may well forecast what is yet to come—real violence involving human blood.

The first was told to me four or five years ago by a high official within one of the Bay Area hospitals' administrative echelons, a woman with impeccable credentials whom I have known for many years and whose integrity I trust.

"I keep on struggling with Irwin Memorial," I told her. "They won't let me arrange for autologous or donor designated blood."

We had discussed this problem before.   When I first realized that HIV might be a threat to transfused patients, I would say to my patients, "Why not give your own blood (termed autologous blood) prior to an operation, or let your family donate their blood for you?" (designated donor blood).

Through my hospital, I had tried many times to get Irwin Memorial to be considerate of patient safety. Each time it was a wrestling match. I might as well have tried to move a mountain. I encountered inertia. I fought bureaucratic resistance. There was unnecessary protocol. There were enormous obstacles, again and again, that the blood banks would put in the way. They didn't want to be bothered with any changes in the way they had always collected blood.

My friend said, "Maybe what you need, Lorraine, is a gun."

She wasn't kidding. It seems that several years ago, a San Francisco police officer was wounded in a shoot-out. His frantic buddies, who ran him to emergency—lights flashing, sirens howling—found out to their dismay about the same red tape, inertia, rhetoric and reticence of the blood bank that I knew all too well.

When the blood bank refused to allow them to donate for their friend, they pulled their guns.

They said, "You *will* take our blood."

The blood bank did.

This was, as far as I know, the first time that Irwin Memorial agreed to let designated donor blood have precedence over general inventory blood.

To my knowledge, this story did not hit the papers.

Just think about the implications: At gunpoint, law-abiding and law-enforcing citizens of San Francisco had to demand a health care safety rule!

Here's story number two.

When Senate investigators several years ago were sent to investigate the safety of the blood supply at the Irwin Memorial Blood Bank, they also came to talk to me. I told them of my futile struggle to stop the blood drives in an area where AIDS was prevalent.

One of the investigators said to me: "Gay terrorism was involved."

According to this official, Irwin Memorial received a threat that if the Castro district was excluded from the blood drives, *there would be a concerted effort on the part of disaffected gays to contaminate the Irwin Memorial blood supply with AIDS on purpose.*

When I think back on all the furor of that summer, this explanation makes a lot of sense to me. What doesn't make much sense is that the government did nothing, after knowing what had occurred. What makes even less sense is that Irwin Memorial caved in.

These two incidents show that we are polarizing. When it comes to AIDS, both sides are willing to let violence speak.

Resorting to violence is not a novel idea.

As long ago as 1983, Robert Schwab, former president of the Texas Human Rights Foundation and a homosexual activist dying of AIDS, had this to bestow on the rest of the world:

> There has come the idea that if research money (for AIDS) is not forthcoming at a certain level by a certain date, all gay males should give blood. . . . Whatever action is required to get national attention is valid. If that includes blood terrorism, so be it.
>
> *Dallas Gay News*
> May 20, 1983

There have been ugly threats like distant thunder, verbally

as well as in print. Often the homosexuals' attitude has been, "I am going to die anyway. I might as well take somebody with me."

It is not a pretty picture.

When I spoke out against the Castro blood drives, I wanted safety for my patients. I knew a few statistics that would have shocked the nation, had they been widely known.

I knew that, based on past records of miscalculation and misinformation, the blood bankers couldn't be trusted.

Here's why:

In the early 1980s, the blood bankers told us that the chances of contracting HIV through blood transfusion was miniscule, the chances were often quoted as one in 1 million.

A few years down the road but still prior to 1985, at which time a blood test became available that tested for *indirect* signs that infection with HIV had occurred—doctors were told in repeated communiques by the blood banks that the risk of AIDS transmission from blood transfusions was somewhere between one in 100,000 and one in 250,000.

"Slim chances," the blood bankers said to the doctors. "The risk is *still* almost nil."

Then evidence began to mount that the risk of infection was "somewhat higher" than commonly believed. We didn't know how much higher, but patients began to fall ill.

Some of us started looking for alternate sources of blood, but nobody knew the actual risk, and the blood banks "discouraged" our challenge. Giving designated donor blood or autologous blood was openly and vigorously resisted by the blood banks. I know, because my patients asked for it, and many times I tried.

But there was protocol. There was "red tape."

The message, then, was clear: Take general inventory blood.

After the spring of 1985, when an HIV antibody test became available, doctors were told that the risk of getting AIDS from a transfusion was now approximately one in 50,000 to one in 100,000. The blood products, the blood bankers told us, were now being treated. The donors were now being carefully screened. There was no need to fret.

In late 1987, it came to light through investigative reporting that those who were operating the voluntary donor blood bank in San Francisco *knew for two years that they had miscalculated the previous risk enormously.*

The risk in one specific year prior to 1985 was not one in 100,000. Not one in 250,000. Not one in 1 million.

It was one in 100!

It was many times that for hemophiliacs who, because of their medical conditions, needed concentrates of blood products from many different donors for their particular transfusions.

Yet the blood banks told no one.

That information was not revealed until two years later. It took headlines to inform the general public and the doctors that *this information had been known for two long years and no one had been notified.*

As reported by *San Francisco Examiner* medical writer Lisa Krieger, it was "fear of AIDS hysteria" that kept the blood risk an official secret.

Here is how Krieger reported this story on November 8, 1987:

> Hospitals and Irwin Memorial Blood Bank knew for several years that The City's blood supply was contaminated by the AIDS virus but thought the risk of infection was too low—and the risk of panic too high—to warn the public.
>
> An estimated 900 Bay Area residents are thought to be infected with the AIDS virus through blood transfusions. They unknowingly could be infecting their sex partners and children, Irwin Memorial Blood Bank data released Friday indicated.
>
> Now, three years after the development of the blood test to detect the AIDS virus, and one year after a study confirmed the presence of viral contamination, hospitals are rushing to warn former patients of possible risks.
>
> "Officials should have acted much sooner," said Dr. Marcus Conant of UC-San Francisco, head of the state task force on the acquired immune deficiency syndrome. "They have been too busy trying to reassure people that there is no problem. There has been downplaying, withholding information and backpedaling from the problem so as not to scare people."
>
> Dr. Herbert A. Perkins, executive director of Irwin, responded, "Everyone was aware that AIDS is carried in blood. People have known that for years." Further action, he said, "could have created hysteria."
>
> In 1982, before the blood test, the chance of getting

one unit of AIDS-contaminated blood was 1 in 100. If several units were needed for major surgery, the risk increased. . . .

The delay in action, people close to the situation believe, was not the result of negligence but uncertainty about *whether the risk was high enough to warrant public alarm.* (Italics added)

Sources said meetings were conducted to discuss the most appropriate action. Officials knew that more than 100,000 Bay Area residents received transfusions during surgery in the high-risk years. To find these people—sending letters, testing and then counseling—could cost thousands of dollars and clog the city's AIDS testing system. . . .

"We are concerned this might cause a large amount of anxiety for a large number of people that we aren't quite ready to handle," Dr. William Hendee, of the American Medical Association, said then.

By May, Irwin had arrived at its own grim conclusions: In 1982, the year of highest risk, 1 in 100 units of blood were infected. In 1981 and 1983, about 1 in 200 units were infected. In 1980 and 1984, 1 in 300 units were infected. *The results were not announced in a press conference. They were posted on the wall of an exhibit hall at the International AIDS Conference in Washington in June.* (Italics added)

Over the next several months, the medical community debated how, and when, to notify the public. They knew that any action taken by The City would be followed elsewhere.

"San Francisco is seen as a model," said Dr. Kathleen

Nolan, a bioethicist at The Hastings Center in Hastings-on-Hudson, N.Y. "There was the risk that a hasty, ill-conceived plan might be mimicked in other places."

The bad news was finally sent to 43 Bay Area hospitals in a letter Aug. 10. Although Irwin Memorial routinely updated hospitals receiving its blood on the number of transfusion-related AIDS fatalities, it had never been so explicit about the extent of contamination. . . .

Hospital officials were shocked. "When we got Irwin's letter, the risk was much higher than I had ever heard before. I hadn't realized that it was nearly that high a risk," said Dr. Steve Darling, chairman of the Blood Utilization Committee of St. Francis Memorial Hospital.

Last week, Kaiser announced it would offer free testing to its 30,000 members who could have been exposed. S.F. General plans to run public service announcements or newspaper advertisements. Ralph K. Davies Medical Center and Marin General also plan to notify former surgical patients about the possibility of infection.

The City and Irwin Memorial are not alone in their dilemma. The Centers for Disease Control estimates that as many as 29,000 Americans may have been infected with the AIDS virus through blood transfusions between 1978 and 1985.

But The City should not have hesitated to alert people, say critics.

"San Francisco should not wait until the federal government issues its recommendations. We should have assessed the problem and moved ourselves," said Conant, the UCSF doctor. "You don't need to wait until you see the actual figures—see the writing on the wall—to do something.

"You don't have to be a mathematical genius to see the implications. As far back as 1982, we knew that it was a blood-borne disease and that many donors were gay," added Conant.

"If we had just said, 'We now know that there is AIDS in blood,' lots of people might have decided against elective surgery. We were not informing them.

"Blood bank officials have been acting as if ignorance is bliss—instead of saying knowledge is strength."

It took almost a decade and unrelenting efforts by Paul Gann, a public figure in California known for property tax reforms and a dying victim of transfusion-transmitted AIDS, to force hospitals and blood banks to abandon lethal practices and inform patients as a matter of routine that there are options other than general inventory blood.

As of January of 1990, the Gann Act makes sure a patient in California has the guarantee that life is valued above protocol.

For many victims, this law has come too late.

My own hospital, San Francisco General, wrote to 17,331 patients who had received transfusions. These patients were told that they faced a "very small risk" of potential AIDS infection. The magnitude of risk, of course, depends on who gets hurt.

There are no numbers anywhere on how many were sentenced to death.

Many of them were my patients.

I myself made several phone calls to patients to tell them that there was a risk they might be infected with AIDS. Those calls were wrenching for me. I can only surmise what the feelings might have been on the other end of the telephone line.

Even so, I commend San Francisco General for notifying patients when they began to see a fuller truth. Not all San Francisco area hospitals, apparently, felt similarly inclined.

To continue the article:

> Even now, knowing the exact risk of exposure, hospitals are reluctant to take similar action. Children's Hospital, St. Francis Memorial Hospital and other medical centers say they will not search for past patients. Instead, *they have asked their doctors to discuss the need for testing when patients come for other treatment.* (Italics added)
>
> "The logistical problems are huge," said Dr. George Rutherford, director of the city Department of Health's AIDS office. "First, you have to find out who received the blood, then you have to find them, test them and counsel them. Some people have moved. Others have died. Each letter could cost hundreds of dollars."
>
> Perkins asked, "Should millions of Americans be sent letters, called in and frightened, costing several hundred million dollars? Is that the best way to stop the AIDS epidemic? Is that the best way to use our money?"

Says Kin Hubbard, "When a fellow says, 'It ain't the money but the principle of the thing,' it's the money."

We may assume that many were infected.

People infected with the HIV virus are mortally ill,

whether they know it or not. They are infectious, whether or not there are symptoms. They have a right to know they are infected with a deadly virus. Their partners have a right to know.

While blood bankers and health officials sat on precedent and protocol so as not to "panic the public," anyone infected through a transfusion could have transmitted the virus.

Those who had sex could have passed AIDS to their sexual partners. Those who became pregnant had a 40 percent chance of giving birth to an AIDS-infected baby. Most of these young victims live less than two years. Some live long enough to enroll in kindergarten.

A very great tragedy caused by the blood banks' patronizing attitude, inertia, and misplaced sense of fiscal conservatism befell the nation's hemophiliacs. This special population became the blood banks' "sitting ducks."

From 1978 through 1985, virtually all hemophiliacs who required the clotting factor were infected through blood bank inventory blood and now face almost certain death.

The following table presents patients with hemophilia who are "believed to be infected with the AIDS virus."

The graph, grim as it is, is deceiving.

We should include their partners. We should add the children who may have been born after transfusion but before diagnosis.

We should add the children who were conceived even after transmission had occurred because the parents were informed, erroneously, that infection did not equal death.

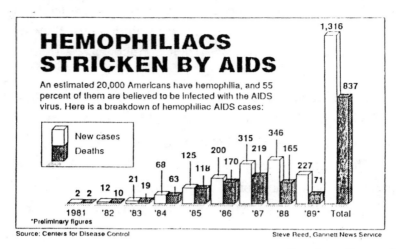

HEMOPHILIACS STRICKEN BY AIDS

An estimated 20,000 Americans have hemophilia, and 55 percent of them are believed to be infected with the AIDS virus. Here is a breakdown of hemophiliac AIDS cases:

New cases
Deaths

1,316
837

2 2 · 12 10 · 21 19 · 68 63 · 125 118 · 200 170 · 315 219 · 346 165 · 227 71

1981 '82 '83 '84 '85 '86 '87 '88 '89* Total

*Preliminary figures

Source: Centers for Disease Control   Steve Reed, Gannett News Service

Stockton Record
April 15, 1990

Hemophilia is a genetic disease where a body cannot, on its own, form the substance that helps it stop bleeding when an injury occurs.

Prior to the availability of Factor VIII, a concentrate that must be pooled from many blood donors, the lifespan of a hemophiliac was short—two or three decades, at most. The development of Factor VIII was hailed as a magnificent scientific breakthrough. It gave a "bleeder" the necessary components to help the blood clot by itself.

It takes many donors to make one routine clotting factor transfusion. Therefore, early in the epidemic before the blood concentrates were treated by a high-heat procedure, a clotting factor transfusion carried many times the chance of passing the virus than did a regular transfusion.

How much of this was known between 1978, when AIDS as a deadly, blood-borne disease first came to the fore, and

1985, when an AIDS antibody test became available?

Consider these facts:

In 1982, both the *Federal Drug Administration* and the *Centers for Disease Control* knew that blood transfusions could transmit the AIDS virus. They also knew with certainty that homosexual men who chose to donate blood were "high risk" in terms of chances of carrying and passing the HIV virus. Virtually all of the diagnosed cases of AIDS were in homosexual men at that time.

The simple task at hand was this: keep homosexual men from giving blood.

There is, of course, no test that tests for homosexuality directly.

There existed a test at that time, however, that could have detected 80 percent of homosexual male blood donors simply because almost all gay males, because of their sexual practices, had anti-hepatitis B core antibody in their blood.

This test was available then, as it is now.

The CDC could have demanded it. The blood banks could have used it. The FDA could have enforced it.

This was three years before an AIDS test was available, which came in use in 1985.

Indeed, the CDC and the FDA told all the blood banks at their national meetings that if they tested with this surrogate test, they could eliminate 80 percent of the AIDS virus from the blood supply by testing who was carrying the anti-hepatitis B core antibody, or in other words, who might be gay.

What happened?

The blood bankers must have reasoned cleverly that if they tested with this test, they would screen out the homosexuals at risk for AIDS, but they would also eliminate a certain percentage of safe donors, people who had had hepatitis, but who were *not* at risk for AIDS.

The estimate was five percent of donors, according to some blood bank minutes I have in my possession.

The blood banks knew that it would take money to recruit new donors to replace them.

It was as plain as that.

Even though the blood bankers are running multi-million dollar businesses, testing was not instituted, apparently because the blood banks chose to "wait and see" what happened to those who received contaminated transfusions rather than to spend the money to recruit new donors.

For three long years, therefore, AIDS-contaminated blood was permitted to become part of the general blood inventory, blood that could have been tested and could have been eliminated.

It infected virtually all the hemophiliacs in the country who needed the clotting factor.

Says Alan Brownstein, executive director of the *National Hemophilia Foundation,* an organization that serves as an advocate for the nation's ravaged hemophiliacs:

"I used to buy a condolence card every time I heard a hemophiliac had died from AIDS. Now I buy those cards by the box."

How could such a holocaust in our midst have happened, with none of us any the wiser?

Consider the chronology as remembered by one

independent blood banker—one of the few courageous voices who spoke out against the mindless tragedy caused by the blood bank industry:

> By November of 1982—through personal conversations, indirect evidence and even public presentations—all blood bankers were aware that the homosexual population was an exceptionally infectious group and must not become blood donors.
>
> Every epidemiologist, public health professional, and most blood bankers had known for a number of years that the homosexual population had an exceptionally high incidence of hepatitis B. They knew persons infected with hepatitis B developed long lasting antibodies against the core antigen of that virus.
>
> It was self-evident that by performing a screening test to detect the presence of anti-(hepaitits) B core antibodies and rejecting the positives, the majority of homosexual donors would be rejected as donors—since a significant number, if not a majority, of homosexuals were infected with AIDS.
>
> It didn't take a mental giant to conclude that the danger of transfusion-transmitted AIDS would be greatly reduced by rejecting anti-hepatitis core positive donors.

In November of 1982, presentations were made at both the ABRA (American Blood Resources Association) and the AABB (American Association of Blood Banks) meetings by the Centers for Disease Control representatives that a variety of potential surrogate tests were available to detect AIDS infection and the AIDS-Related Complex (ARC) condition.

Three of those stood out in particular—the anti-core test, the T4/T8 lymphocyte ratio, and the condition known as lymphocytopenia. Any prudent person would have implemented one of those 3 tests as soon as possible.

Hesitation to implement was due to fear of losing "good" donors. There were estimates that as many as 5 percent of otherwise acceptable donors might have antibodies against hepatitis B core and yet not carry AIDS.

A large percentage of homosexuals, particularly sexually active homosexuals, would be detected by one of these tests, and these very persons would be significantly dangerous donors.

A choice existed between rejecting an unknown but large number of infectious donors while at the same time losing as many as 5% percent of "good" donors—or taking the chance of releasing infectious blood. (Italics added)

I have no personal knowledge of this being discussed in the Joint Committee, but I find it inconceivable that it was not. It boiled down to one simple decision by the blood bankers: "Do we want to institute a surrogate test that will probably reject 70—80% of the AIDS carriers—but in doing so will "lose" as many as 5 percent of otherwise normal, healthy donors?"

The alternative was: "Take a chance; don't perform a surrogate test; let the blood go through and see what happens."

In other terms, take a chance with the life of the recipients of blood products or work harder to recruit and make up for the 5 percent of "lost" donors.

You and I would say that the economics of such a decision are overwhelmingly in favor of working harder at recruiting. The ethics or morality of doing otherwise, I think, are open to independent judgment.

In January of 1983 the *National Hemophilia Foundation* demanded a conference of all responsible parties. Their own medical advisory board made recommendations to protect their constituency.

In that same month, the *Centers for Disease Control* called a conference of all interested organizations. A variety of recommendations, opinions, and data were presented—including a re-presentation of the November 1982 surrogate test data (data regarding testing for anti-hepatitis B-core antibody).

The results of this meeting were rapidly transmitted to every single blood banker in the United States through all four trade associations representing them.

This immediately became the overwhelming subject of discussion among blood bankers both verbally and in writing and remains so today.

Any blood banker who claims he was not knowledgeable of the problem and the logical, though partial, solution in the spring of 1983 had to have been deaf, dumb, blind *and* dead.

We may assume that most blood bankers were then, and are still, alive and well, which can't be said, unfortunately, of the majority of our nation's hemophiliacs.

While in America we, with our clotting factors were

infecting the entire hemophiliac population, Germany, as reported by the *New England Journal of Medicine*[1], did not infect their hemophiliacs, although they bought much of their blood from us.

I thought that was a puzzling mystery.   I called up a hospital blood bank colleague, and I asked her.

She said to me: "You always ask the right questions."

I said: "Germany must have been processing their clotting factor differently from the way we were processing ours. I am sure their greater safety record wasn't just coincidence."

As it turns out, yes. There was a reason. *Apparently, their way of treatment was more expensive.*

This knowledge must have been available in the United States. It is hard to believe it was not.

Our blood bankers, for reasons best known to them, did not choose to use the more expensive procedure and, therefore, lives were lost.

"But that was then," says the man in the street. "In the beginning, we didn't know these frightening statistics about AIDS and the dangers of blood transfusions. But now the blood is being tested."

That is true. Now the blood is being tested, and it is much safer than it was five years ago.

It is safer, but not safe. AIDSpeak won't make that distinction.

The blood banks are not testing for the virus. There is no routinely available blood test that targets the virus directly.

They are testing for the antibodies to the virus.

For any testing to be meaningful, the body must have had

time to have reacted to the virus. It then develops antibodies. Just as a fire needs time to develop, so does a body's immune system need time to react to virus invasion. Once it reacts, we can detect that HIV is there.

It says nothing, however, about how long it may have been smoldering quietly.

Some infections "take" quicker than others. Some immune reactions may take several years before antibodies develop.

This period is called the "negative window" period, when an infected person, asymptomatic, could potentially spread the disease by donating blood. The donor wouldn't know. The blood banks wouldn't know. The blood test is negative.

We used to think that the time period between infection and antibody production was something like three months. Many articles for the past decade have "documented" staunchly that this period, on the average, was about twelve weeks between exposure and antibody presence.

These calculations were done, repeated, and statistically "verified" because the disease was so new.

Those were the infections that "showed."

We didn't know about the ones that didn't show as yet. We didn't know that antibodies took their time and could not always be detected.

Based on that "knowledge" and vociferous AIDSpeak propaganda, it is believed to this day by many health care workers, even in high echelons, that the risk of infection by asymptomatic carriers wishing to donate their blood is around 1 for every 40,000 units of donated blood.

That ratio was based on calculations of a 3-month negative window.

We now know that antibody formation may take as long as three-and-a-half years.

I submit to any reasonable person that the risks of "negative window" exposure will have to be recalculated in light of what we now know.

Even making allowances for the crime of *omission* due to partial knowledge, a concession we really can't afford to make since lives are being lost through negligence, there is the crime of *commission*: release of potentially dangerous blood because of accident or human error.

As reported in the *American Medical News,* in October of 1988:

> The American Red Cross has signed an agreement with the Food and Drug Administration to improve the safety of its blood banks after learning it had mistakenly released 2,420 blood products.
>
> "Most mistakes involved donations that tested negative for AIDS, but for various reasons were not in compliance with Red Cross or FDA directives that require such donations to be quarantined and/or destroyed," said Victor W. Schmitt, vice president, Blood Services of the Red Cross at Washington, D. C., national headquarters.
>
> An example is blood from a donor who falsely tests positive for a blood disease and gives blood again, he said. Under FDA rules, the blood cannot be released, even if it tests negative for AIDS and hepatitis B.
>
> "The most serious finding was that 518 blood products had been released before all record checks or testing had

been completed," Schmitt said.

Was this an isolated "human error" committed by one careless blood bank? Not according to the *AIDS Litigation Reporter*:

> Announcing on September 14 the completion of a six month audit of its own operational procedures, *the American Red Cross has uncovered flaws blamed for the distribution of more than 2,400 units of tainted blood through 30 of its 56 regional blood centers during the study period.* (Italics added) . . .
>
> Almost 75% of the blood units mistakenly distributed tested AIDS-positive or came from donors who had previously tested positive. The remainder of the blood was from persons who had tested positive for any of a number of infectious diseases, including hepatitis. Red Cross officials say much of the blood in question came from the "false positive" category which should have been discarded but was not, due to a computer filing error.

Such "errors" make me edgy.

As a trauma surgeon in the trenches of a city with the highest per capita AIDS count in the U.S., I don't have a lot of confidence in so-called "safety statistics" when it comes to blood from our blood banks—banks that are run by officials who think nothing of holding blood drives in the Castro. "An appeaser," said Winston Churchill, "is one who feeds a crocodile, hoping it will eat him last."

It's not just Irwin Memorial. It's not just San Franciso.

Not even just California and New York. We have a national blood exchange. We still import some of our blood from Mexico and other countries with less than adequate testing. As this book is written, we have an Associated Press report out of Chicago that blood banks aren't squeamish generally as to the populations from whom they get their blood:

> Despite efforts to discourage them, drug abusers who are infected with the AIDS virus still are selling blood plasma to commercial collection centers, and more needs to be done to stop them, a study says.
>
> But a spokesman for plasma collection centers says they are doing a good job of excluding such donors and keeping the AIDS infection out of blood products.
>
> "The current products that are out there are considered to be 100 percent safe," said James Reilly, spokesman for the American Blood Resources Association.
>
> The study found that more than 23 percent of 2,921 intravenous drug abusers contacted in the Baltimore area in 1988 and 1989 said they had sold plasma or donated blood after they began injecting illegal drugs.
>
> Tests revealed 24.1 percent of those contacted were infected with HIV, the AIDS virus.

> *Los Angeles Times*
> April 25, 1990

"The greatest evil," says C.S. Lewis, "is not done in those sordid dens of crime that Dickens loved to paint... it is conceived and moved, seconded, carried and minuted in clean, carpeted, warmed and well-lighted offices by quiet men with white collars and cut fingernails and smooth-shaven cheeks who do not need to raise their voices."

4

The Myth of Self-Deferral

"The FDA did not require an AIDS test on donated blood until January 5, 1988, almost three years after the first test for detecting AIDS antibodies in blood came into use in March 1985."

"Between 1987 and 1988, the number of recalls of suspect blood almost tripled."

"For at least a year, people who had tested positive for the deadly AIDS virus were allowed to walk the streets of Philadelphia without knowing it. They had sold their blood plasma to the Community Bank and Plasma Center. . . The Center tested the blood for the AIDS virus and until 1987 notified in writing anyone who tested positive, according to a company executive. But that year, the Center stopped mailing these notifications after a city-funded AIDS group objected to the way it was being done."

"There is no federal regulation requiring blood banks to

notify donors who test positive for AIDS. The Food and Drug Administration, the federal agency responsible for the safety of the American blood supply, recommends notifying donors but leaves the decision up to the blood banks and plasma centers."

"From March 1988 to March 1989, blood banks and commercial plasma centers had to recall nearly 100,000 blood components and medicines made from blood that had been erroneously released, FDA records show."

"In this marketplace, blood, a vital resource, gets less government protection than grapes or poultry or pretzels. Dog kennels in Pennsylvania are inspected more frequently than blood banks."

> Quotes from the Philadelphia Inquirer,
> Sept 24-28—Five-part Series on Blood Banks
> Gilbert M. Gaul, Reporter

Much political hay has been cut with the cheerful assertion that those who should not give their blood in blood bank drives will be responsible enough *not to want to do so.*

The AIDSpeak term is "self-deferral."

Self-deferral, unfortunately, does not work, for psychological as well as for practical reasons.

Imagine that you are a willing female donor and what is called a "low-risk" donor. You walk into a blood bank drive, propelled by the purest of motives, and you are handed a paper that informs you, in part:

People who are at risk for AIDS must not donate blood.

If any of the following descriptions apply to you,
Do Not Donate Blood

* If you have AIDS or have tested positive for HIV antibody.

* If you are a male who has had sex with another male EVEN ONCE since 1977.

* If you inject yourself with drugs not prescribed by a physician or have done so in the past, EVEN ONCE.

* If you emigrated to the United States from Haiti or Sub-Saharan Africa including islands off the coast of Africa.

* If you are a hemophiliac who has received clotting factor concentrates.

* If you have had sex with anyone described in the above categories, EVEN ONCE.

* If you have engaged in prostitution since 1977 or had sex within the last 12 months with someone who has, EVEN ONCE.

Your blood will be tested for:

* AIDS
* Hepatitis
* Syphilis
* HTLV

You will be notified if you are found ineligible to donate blood because of a positive test result.

You read that, and your heart starts pounding. Although you were always careful, you're not so sure your partners were, because, now working backwards, you realize that it is 1990, and they are talking thirteen years.

You were discreet, and you had principles, but who's to say what might have happened thirteen years ago in someone else's life that you were not aware of?

So here you are, thirteen years later, with this rather threatening piece of paper in your hand that tells you that you might be punished for somebody else's reckless behavior. To say the least, you had expected some discreet and dignified treatment. Resentment builds and defense mechanisms kick in.

You swallow, determined to give blood. You push away painful misgivings as you sit down and open what is known as the "self-deferral" questionnaire that will help the blood banks determine if you are a "safe" and trustworthy donor. After writing down your social security number, along with name, address, telephone number, birthdate, age and occupation, you start answering 37 questions, but not before you ask yourself aggressively: "What's all this fuss about confidentiality? Isn't my donation supposed to be confidential? Where is this information going? Into some government computer bank?"

Your choice is "Yes" or "No."

1. Do you have AIDS, AIDS Related Complex (ARC) or a positive test for the AIDS virus?

2. Are you a male who has had sex with another male EVEN ONCE since 1977?

3. Ever injected yourself with drugs EVEN ONCE or had sex with someone who has EVEN ONCE?

4. Have you emigrated to the United States from Sub-Saharan Africa or Haiti?

5. Are you a hemophiliac who has received clotting factor concentrates?

6. Since 1977 have you had sexual contact EVEN ONCE or otherwise been in contact with any body fluids of a person described in the above categories?

You say to yourself, feeling even more threatened: "I just *answered* these questions!   Who designed this impossible form?" However, you came here to donate blood and donate blood you will and therefore, you push on.

7. Are you a woman who has been artificially inseminated since 1977?

8. Have you engaged in prostitution since 1977 or had sex within the last 12 months with someone who has EVEN ONCE?

9. Have you ever been tested for AIDS anywhere other than at Irwin?

10. Ever had unexplained night sweats, fevers, weight loss, persistent diarrhea or persistent cough?

11. Ever had lymphadenopathy (swollen glands) or Kaposi's Sarcoma (unexplained purple spots on skin) or thrush (white spots in the mouth)?

12. Are you donating to be tested for AIDS?

13. Do you understand that a person infected with the AIDS virus can feel well and show no symptoms of infection?

14. Ever had yellow jaundice, hepatitis, a positive blood test for hepatitis or any liver disease?

15. Been exposed to anyone with yellow jaundice or hepatitis in the last 12 months?

16. Received hepatitis B immune globulin in the past 12 months?

17. Ever received blood or blood plasma transfusions or blood injections?

18. Received any inoculations or vaccinations in the past month?

19. Been treated for rabies in the past 12 months?

20. Had tattoos, ears pierced, acupuncture, electrolysis or any other skin piercing in the past 12 months?

21. Had malaria or taken anti-malarial medication in the past three years?

22. Been outside USA in the past 3 years?

23. Ever been pregnant or pregnant now?

24. Ever been seriously ill?

25. Have you had brucellosis, relapsing fever or babesiosis?

26. Been hospitalized or had surgery in the past 12 months?

27. Ever had blood abnormalities, bleeding tendency or cancer?

28. Ever had a venereal disease?

29. Ever had a heart or lung disease, chest pain, shortness of breath, tuberculosis, asthma or diabetes?

30. Had any history of convulsions, seizures or fainting spells?

31. Taken aspirin, aspirin products or anti-inflammatories in the past 72 hours? (Not necessarily a reason for refusal)

32. Taken any medications in the past month (including Accutane)?

33. Any known allergies?

34. Had a tooth pulled or mouth surgery in the past 72 hours?

35. Ever been refused as a blood donor or donated blood in the past 8 weeks?

36. Ever been treated with growth hormone made from human pituitary glands?

37. Do you have an infection or feel ill today?

The print is small. The language is intimidating. Some of the questions seem irrelevant or more than just faintly intrusive. No. You have *never* been treated for rabies!

Some of the questions seem picky.

You did have night sweats once—but that was the flu, wasn't it? And you did travel outside the USA, but that was Canada—still on the Continent. The point is that *you answer as you think you should—with as much candor as you can.*

You sign your signature below the statement verifying that you understand you should not donate blood if you have any reason to believe that you have been exposed to AIDS or hepatitis. You are *fairly* sure about AIDS, but hepatitis? And what about brucellosis, relapsing fever and babesiosis?

You take your questionnaire to the nurse. She sits there, looking bored, having watched you all the while because there aren't all that many donors present and she has nothing else to do.

She is a bit partitioned off, but it is not a fully -enclosed cubicle: Anybody in the donor hall could listen in on what she says to you or what you might tell her.

The nurse scans your answers. She never once makes eye contact. She says softly: "I am going to ask you the first 13 questions *again.*"

You say "No" thirteen times—feeling very foolish now.

You came here with all the best intentions. You thought that your donation made a difference! Are you here to be grilled for the sins of yourself or your partner(s)?

And the nurse—she doesn't like this any more than you do. She lets that be known by her body language: It's like having to disrobe, isn't it? Necessary, but embarrassing. It's just a mere formality. She speaks in a soft monotone. *No way* does *she* imply that she thinks you are a prostitute, a Haitian, a homosexual, a heroin fiend, or a hemophiliac.

Duty dispensed, she pricks your finger. She says your iron count is fine. She takes your temperature and your pulse and hands you back your form, along with a card that has two little stickers relating to the blood that you will give.

One says: "Use." The other says: "Don't use."

"Go over there," she says. "Pull off one of the stickers and put it on this spot."

By now, you feel uncomfortable, indeed because you know she knows, and so does everybody else in that big hall, for people had their ears cocked—that you have fibbed a little, if not a lot, not necessarily about yourself but maybe about your partner(s). Since you were not celibate between some thirteen years ago and now, the truth be told, there was somebody in your past who could have fallen into one or more of the suspicious categories.

You don't think so, however. You are in good health now.

You are older now, and wiser, and there were never, to your knowledge, any serious repercussions. You never once, in your entire life, were forced to go to County Health to ask them to clean up your act.

An acquaintance of mine described this experience because she recently gave blood at the dubious Castro location. She happens to be one of the most conservative women I know. She is a rather brainy woman, discriminating in her relationships. But she was not so sure at all—in the strictest sense of the questions that she answered—that she qualified as a "safe donor."

The point of this vignette is not to say she may have been at risk. The point is that this woman did not tell the entire truth, the whole truth and nothing but the truth—and neither would most people. Pertaining to their sexual history, most people do not tell the truth. They don't even know the truth about their partners. This donor "reasoned" with herself. If anyone's blood was safe, hers would be safe. She wasn't going to allow herself or anybody else to think otherwise. She had come to give blood, and that's what she did. She gave blood.

She walked out thinking how many donors with pasts more checkered than hers might have lied with equal *chutzpah.*

As a screening instrument, the blood bank's questionnaire and the follow-up "verbal screening" are worthless.

As for my friend, the screening rules were so restrictive and embarassing the Pope might not have passed. And never once was there a dignified "way out," had she run scared and wanted to back out because she might have thought that her blood was compromised. There was no effort whatsoever to get only simon-pure blood. The questionnaire and "follow-up screening" by the nurse were mere formalities, designed to cover legal liability.

As the Castro controversy proved to me more than two years ago, the blood banks as well as special interest groups become choleric if anyone suggests there might be motives other than pure altruism that might make a donor want to give blood.

A "questionable donor," it has been repeatedly claimed, if given a chance to withdraw discreetly, will certainly jump at the chance. A donor is given an opportunity to screen himself out—to disqualify himself by "donating" his sample to "research."

But does it work in practice? No. At least at the Castro location, there was not even an attempt to encourage my friend to withdraw. The self-deferral form will not stop anyone. That puts the burden of proof on the laboratory testing itself.

I would like to juxtapose the experience above with the findings of a research article published less than seven months before in the *New England Journal of Medicine*.[1]

The statistical parameters of this study would be beyond the interest of the casual reader. The intent here is merely to give a flavor of what researchers find when they dig into donor motives and subsequent results. These excerpts from that article have been selected to enhance clarity:

> Of 693,000 volunteer blood donors in Washington, D. C., who were screened for infection with human immunodeficiency virus type 1 (HIV-1) from July 1985 through December 1988, 284 tested positive on both enzyme immunoassay and Western blot assay. (The screening test and the more definitive test, respectively, for HIV)

> Despite the use of questionnaires to identify those at high risk for exposure to HIV, some persons who have engaged in high-risk behavior continue to donate blood.

> The enzyme immunoassay used as the screening test does not detect all infected donors, and the transmission of HIV by blood products found to be negative for HIV

antibody has been documented.

Of the 128 men (in the group who tested positive on Western blot assay), 83 percent had engaged in sexual activity with another man, and 3 percent had used intravenous drugs.

The majority of the 28 women who tested positive on Western blot (86 percent) had strong evidence supporting heterosexual exposure, that was documented in one-third by HIV-testing of the sexual partner and inferred in the others from a history of sexual contact with a man in a high-risk group. In two women and one man, exposure by blood transfusion was proved.

Despite having read the literature on voluntary self-exclusion provided at the blood center, the majority of these donors did not believe that their activities had placed them personally at risk for exposure to HIV. In addition, although alternative testing sites were available, donating blood in order to obtain HIV testing was not uncommon.

All 33 donors exposed to HIV through hetero-sexual activity were unaware that their behavior had placed them at risk for HIV infection, including those who knew before donation that their partners had used intravenous drugs (33 percent) or engaged in prostitution (26 percent).

The results of our study suggest that current

measures for donor education and screening are not uniformly effective in eliminating from the donor pool people at high risk . *The majority of our HIV-infected donors understood the definition of high-risk behavior but did not view themselves as having engaged in such behavior.* (Italics added)

Even more disturbing, a large proportion donated specifically in order to discover the results of HIV-testing. Furthermore, less than 5 percent understood the purpose of the post-donation confidential unit-exclusion system and would have designated their units as solely for research.

The majority of the donors exposed through hetero-sexual contact were unaware that high-risk behavior in their partners had placed them at risk for HIV infection, and they had no basis for voluntary self-exclusion.

It does not take a statistician to conclude that unsafe donors permitted to have access to the general blood supply pose at least a theoretical danger to the recipient of a blood transfusion.

People who come to give blood to a blood bank location will want to give blood and will do so.

Common-sense reasons why self-deferral does not work might be:

Some people donate in order to have themselves tested for HIV or other venereal diseases under conditions of anonymity and at no cost to them.

Some might seek reassurance. Donors might need to tell themselves they understand the definition of "high risk" but it does not apply to them.

Some think that monogamous sex puts them outside the risk factors.

Work places may put pressure on people to donate blood who should not have to do so. A closet homosexual who has a promotion pending and a boss who is an ardent Jerry Falwell fan might not have much incentive to refuse.

Some larger corporations offer "perks," such as a day off work for donating blood. Some people might need a day off to go shopping or run errands.

Some people have poor vision and cannot read the very fine print of the intimidating self-deferral form.

Thanks to our public schools, some people cannot read.

Some gays have threatened to infect the blood supply on purpose unless certain medical or political demands are being met.

What is the solution for safer blood in light of inadequate screening, testing, the "negative window factor," and import of blood from sources that cannot be easily tracked?

A good way to start might be through enlightened consumerism. Here are a few suggestions.

One very simple way of making the blood supply safer is to solicit women's blood. As has been documented, women's blood is as much as nine times safer than men's.[1]

According to Leslie Dutton, President of the American Association of Women who testified to the President's AIDS Commission, her organization offered to be actively involved in recruiting women donors. She also wanted gender-labeling, to give patients additional safety. Not only was this not done, but there was actual resistance and suppression of evidence that female blood is safer than male blood. Her testimony was eliminated from the AIDS Commission's final document.

Said Dutton in a telephone interview: "The bottom line is money."

Patients need to know that there are various ways they can protect themselves with safer blood than the blood banks can presently provide.

The safest blood, of course, is your own.

Thanks to the tireless efforts of my friend and fellow trooper, Paul Gann, California now has a law that guarantees you will have options. Your doctor must inform you that, at your request and prior to an elective operation, your blood can be drawn at safe intervals, refrigerated or frozen and held until you need it.

This procedure by which your own pre-operative blood is set aside specifically for you is called "autologous donation." Obviously, this option might not always be available if, for example, you are injured in an accident on the East Coast, while your autologous donation is stored on the West Coast and can't be flown in fast enough to aid an emergency situation. Nonetheless you should know that there are new privately funded blood banks being opened that with advanced technology can store several frozen pints of your own blood for many years.

Competition by these blood storage banks has not been welcomed by the American Red Cross and other regular blood banks.

At present, you have two choices other than homologous blood (general blood bank inventory blood): first a technique called the cell-saver procedure and second, if there is time, designated donor blood.

Although the cell saver technology is not new it is fairly expensive and requires a specially trained technician, which adds further to the cost. The equipment for this procedure can also be leased by a hospital. We at SF General have used it regularly for four or five years. It works much like a vacuum cleaner by sucking up blood from the operation site that might otherwise be lost, purifying it, repackaging it, and putting it back into your body. It can't be used, however, for cancer operations, infections, or contaminated wounds. This procedure is less expensive than taking a risk with someone else's blood that may not be safe and should be mandatory in cases of extensive blood loss.

Your second option is to ask for designated donor blood which is blood from people you have reason to believe would be safe donors for you or your loved ones.

You don't have any guarantees with designated donor blood. If someone infected with HIV in your workplace, for example, were to receive a call to donate blood for a close friend in an emergency, it would be virtually impossible to deny such an emotional request.

In these times of widespread secrecy pertaining to the

virus, and given the long incubation period for AIDS, designated donor blood may or may not be safer than general inventory blood. It boils down, say the blood banks, to a matter of personal judgment.

I still say it is safer if you know the donor well. Immediate family members, particularly women, would be a very good bet for most Americans not yet infected with AIDS.

There are vested interests that will tell you that you do not need to take that step, especially if there is money to be made in the sale and distribution of blood. There will be statistics to back up that assertion. An Irwin Memorial Blood Bank study,[2] published some 18 months after screening for the HIV virus started, stated its procedures and findings as follows:

Our designated donor program began on June 1, 1984. Prior to this date, each designated donation request had to be initiated by the patient's physician. A blood bank physician screened each request, explained the steps taken to insure blood safety, the 48 hour minimum time frame, and alternative sources of blood, i. e., autologous transfusion, to the patient's physician. If the designated donations were accepted, the donor could only donate at the main headquarters center in San Francisco or at the Shasta Center in Redding Monday through Friday. Red cells were the only products available. . . .

The original protocol contained many obstacles that we felt would discourage the use of the program. We found that patients wanted the program whether or not the obstacles were there, so we began to streamline the protocol to make it easier for patients as well as the blood bank employees.

Please note the initial "red tape" and admitted deliberate attempts by the blood banks to "discourage the use of the program." Only after patients and doctors both kept demanding alternate blood did Irwin Memorial change its procedures. The "conclusion," however, was still in favor of general inventory donorship:

> Irwin Memorial Blood Bank, after drawing and processing over 11,000 designated donors, feels that potential patients and their families are able to recruit donors who are *as safe but not demonstrably more safe* than volunteer, homologous donors recruited by our donor recruiters.

This paper looks at three sub-groups: first-time donors, many-times donors and designated donors. Statistics indicate across the board that the designated donors are no safer than the blood bank donors for hepatitis. *But they are safer for AIDS.*

This finding is presented in the graph, but it is never mentioned in the article. I don't know if this difference is statistically significant or not, and the researcher does not say that it is not.

I looked at the graph and I wondered. Why did the authors not mention it?

To me it didn't seem to make much sense that designated donor blood was considered no safer than the regular blood supply. If my children had been unfortunate enough to have been in an accident, I know that I would have wanted them to have my mother's, my aunt's or even my best friend's blood rather than blood that came from the Castro. And so, I believe, would most people.

But in a quirky way, statistically, the findings may be true because volunteer donors who give over and over again are tested many times, and therefore, by definition, are seen as "low risk" people.

This study, however, does not differentiate demographically and socioeconomically. It is talking about blood in all spectrums, including blood from your family that might be very safe compared to blood from a drug addict's friends. Naturally a drug addict's friend's blood isn't going to be as safe as your family's blood, but if somebody takes a statistical average of the general population, there will be no "significant difference."

Statistics, said a pundit, are like bikinis. What they reveal is exciting, but what they hide is vital.

One final word: there is so much yet to be done in tightening our safety standards not just for blood banks but for bone banks, semen banks, and tissue and organ transplant banks as well.

I was a member of the Centers for Disease Control Committee in August of 1988 that wrote the first AIDS guidelines for bone banks. By then, we had our first *known* casualty—a young patient who had become infected from a bone graft.

"But guidelines should have been written," I argued, "more than four years ago!"

Apparently, it took a revelation and a "dead body" to

produce a simple protocol. This young woman nurse, age 23, had idiopathic scoliosis—curvature of the spine. During a spine fusion, she had received no blood transfusions, but she had received bone, later found to have come from a drug addict, a donor who was subsequently found to have AIDS. Two years later, the woman was also diagnosed with AIDS. "Every doctor in the world," I pushed on, "knows that the substance that nourishes a bone is blood. Did it not dawn on you that if blood transmitted HIV, then bone, semen, connective tissue, tendons and all organs should also transmit HIV?" Blank stares.

I said stubbornly, "I'd like to have an answer. Why are we writing these regulations five years after the fact? You knew in 1983 that blood transmitted the disease. Common sense would tell you that this would happen. Any body tissue that contains blood ought to have been automatically suspect."

"But we've never seen it happen," they responded.

The consensus in that CDC room was sheer textbook AIDSpeak: *to infer transmission without evidence would have been unwarranted and highly suspect speculation unworthy of this august fellowship.*

I said: "I'm a trauma surgeon, and there are certain things that I can logically infer at no risk to my competence or veracity."

Let me give you an example. In the past, I have seen people who have fallen twelve stories from the Bank of America Building. Chances are, that when I saw them, they were dying if not dead. But if someone falls twelve stories from another building, say the Transamerica Pyramid Building, lands on the cement, and is brought in to me in bits and pieces, I would not stand here, saying, "What a surprise! Who would have thought that fellow would have died from that fall!" I would have known from past experience that if somebody fell twelve stories from any building, the consequence would be grave injury if not death.

Although inferences such as these are obvious and legitimate in medicine, the Centers for Disease Control has chosen not to make them, demonstrating again and again their lack of courage and their capitulation to political pressures at the expense of human lives.

5

The Epidemic Explodes

"Many gays reject morality, offering any one of a variety of reasons, rational and emotional, for doing so. But there's a simpler, darker reason why many gays choose to live without morality: as ideologies go, amorality is damned convenient. And the mortal enemy of that convenience is the value judgment.

It quickly became clear to us that urban gays assumed a general consensus to the effect that everyone has the right to behave just as he pleases. . . Everyone was to decide what was "right for him"—in effect, to make up the rules as he went along. In fact, they boiled down to a single axiom: I can do whatever I want, and you can go to perdition. . . .

We found that in the gay press this doctrine had hardened into stone. The more outrageous the behavior, the more it was to be seen as "celebrating our unique sensibility and culture": the less ethically defensible, the less one was to feel entitled to speak out against it, lest one be accused of attempting to resurrect that bugbear, "traditional morality."

After the Ball[1]

pp 291-93.

The preceding passage is taken from a well-written book by two Harvard-trained social scientists, Marshall Kirk and Hunter Madsen, both of them homosexual. The book was given to me as a present by a special friend whom I shall call Mark in this chapter. Mark is gay also.

I will rely on Mark's and on Kirk and Madsen's observations of the gay scene of the past two decades as backdrop for the things I have to say. I want to speak freely, scalpel in hand, of the gay community's involvement in, and contribution to, the mind-boggling, health-shattering explosion of AIDS. As Kirk and Madsen put it so eloquently, "AIDS rode into town this morning, and soon it will be high noon."

You have, no doubt, heard the illuminating tale of three blind men who felt different anatomical parts of an elephant. One thought that the trunk was the elephant and described the elephant in terms of its trunk characteristics. Another thought that the tail was more descriptive of the entire elephant. A third insisted loudly that its beautiful tusks were what really defined elephant essence, and everybody else's mental picture of the elephant was wrong.

The point of the story, of course, is limited grasp, biased thinking, and skewed reasoning that spring from a narrow perspective. Often missed when this story is told is the reality, however, that the trunk, the tusks and the tail are *all* part of the elephant. They make up the elephant. To explain them away is limited grasp, biased thinking, and skewed reasoning, too.

Therefore, without apologies, I will describe the parts of the allegorical creature that I have come to know. As a doctor working in a trauma hospital in San Francisco, I want to speak of injuries resulting from gay sex, both to the individuals directly involved and now, via AIDS, to us all.

I know that there are many other parts to the proverbial

elephant that I am not describing. I leave description of those parts to others to have their say their way.

Here's mine.

In San Francisco, tourists can buy themselves T-shirts that say, "I'm a PWA," Person With AIDS.

Why not PWS, PWG, or PWH—Person With Syphilis, Person With Gonorrhea, or Person With Herpes?

That kind of flaunting is uncalled for. It offends the sensibilities. It brings on a visceral response. It is the kind of irresponsibility that non-gay America sees, the kind that lies down on the Golden Gate Bridge, kicking and screaming much like a three-year-old, demanding "adult's rights."

The kind that stomps, whistles, shrieks and throws paperballs at Louis B. Sullivan, a respected United States Cabinet member, addressing an international audience concerned with the most serious health care problem our times have ever faced.

The kind that shouts down scientists who work to find a cure.

The kind that behaves like nothing more than spoiled children.

The kind whose behavior was reported in an article that came across my desk a few months ago in the form of a University of California, San Francisco publication:

4 Arrested, 39 Cited At UCSF Men's Room

Investigation of a series of thefts led police at the University of California, San Francisco (UCSF) medical center to arrest four men for lewd conduct in a campus

restroom. Another 39 people were stopped by police
and given warnings for loitering in the area. . . .Instead
of catching a thief, however, plainclothes officers observed
sexual acts and much cruising, loitering and solicitation,
police said.

"We began to make arrests to give notice that this
had to stop," said Joseph Cowan, UCSF assistant
chancellor for legal affairs. He said that UCSF officials
had known that "this was going on for some time". . . .

David Goldberg, of the Campus Gay Men's
Support Group, was critical of the university for
acting so suddenly.

"That particular bathroom has been notorious
for years," he said, "but *for the university to up and
do something without fair warning is ridiculous.*" (Italics
added).

I agree with a wise man named Oliver Herford, who said,
"If some people got their rights, they would complain of being
deprived of their wrongs."

That kind of behavior is at the very least discourteous, and
at the most, repugnant. What about the rights of other people
in the bathroom? Few heterosexuals would need to be
reminded that sexual activity requires privacy, and that our
public restrooms, parks, and bookstores are not suitable to the
pursuit of quick and anonymous sex.

What translates to me as a doctor when I am informed of
behavior as described above is *the evidence that immaturity and
irresponsibility are costly. What homosexuals do, and how
they think about their actions, cannot be had for free. It's
costing all of us. It's costing human lives.*

Long before we knew of AIDS, a very well-known San Francisco health official repeatedly warned the gay community of San Francisco that there would be very serious consequences to traumatic sex with countless numbers of partners. The oft-repeated argument that gays did not know about AIDS and, hence, fell innocent victim to AIDS, is simply not a fact.

They were told repeatedly, in many more ways than one. They were warned that if this behavior continued they could not remain healthy. Something disastrous would happen.

It did.

If you go by AIDSpeak etiquette, you go by certain rules. One of them demands that you must always preface speculation about the origins and spread of AIDS by stating firmly for the record that AIDS does not discriminate, that AIDS is not gender-specific nor sex orientation specific. Another demands that a person with AIDS is not responsible for having the disease and should have no guilt. Given unfortunate exposure, it strikes both gays and straights.

Indeed it does, as does a fire, once set and left unchecked.

The point that must be made is not about the nature of the fire. Where it first came from is an open question. I speak about conditions, attitudes and practices within the gay community that have managed to fuel the fire. I speak about conditions, attitudes and practices still standing in the way when people risk their lives to try to put it out.

When I speak about the gay community and its contribution to the AIDS epidemic, I speak about male homosexuality. There have been cases of lesbians giving AIDS to each other, but they are rare, and generally, the lesbian community is probably one of the least affected and safest subgroups in the AIDS epidemic. It has been my observation as well, as I have watched the gay and lesbian scene in San Francisco, that lesbian love is different in kind and in degree from the attraction that men have for each other. Lesbians can form monogamous relationships that are supportive, nurturing, long-lasting, respectful of each other, and generally not harmful physically.

The same is not true, as a rule, of gay males.

I bring a medical judgment to male homosexuality. Morality, like art, consists in drawing the line somewhere. As a physician, I will now draw that line.

I recently heard about a rather famous male actor, you may have, too, for the story came over the wire, who had a dead gerbil removed from his rectum. That is not normal sexual behavior. That is not a "variation" of lifestyle. It is depraved and self-abusive sex.

It has been my observation during 15 years as a doctor in one of the world's most-frequented trauma hospitals that much of gay sex is of the harmful, sadistic and/or masochistic variety. Gays hurt each other. They also hurt themselves.

One does not have to moralize about the rightness or wrongness of gay male sexual behavior. I don't believe that God singles out gay men for punishment. Nature imposes its own penalty. As a physician, I know very well that if we abuse our bodies we will get sick and possibly die.

There are very serious health consequences to abusive and

self-abusive sexual behavior. Gay males as a rule have been abusive to themselves and to their partners to a degree that is incomprehensible within the heterosexual world. Gay bathhouses have become the well-known dens of death from which AIDS has sprung like a specter straight out of hell.

A good place to start discussing abusive gay sex long practiced in the gay bathhouses would be with drugs. Says Mark, now in his fifties, who was there when Gay Liberation came to San Francisco:

> The 1970s produced a period when gay people truly could do practically anything they wanted to—have sex in the parks, such as Buena Vista and Lands End, have sex in certain men's rooms at key high rise buildings downtown during lunch break, and generally have 24-hour non-stop sex.
>
> This was brought on in large part by two factors: the gay liberation, with the discovery of voting power held by the gay population of San Francisco, and also by the development and acceptance of drugs in the gay community at large.
>
> In 1965, poppers (amyl nitrate) became the "in" drug among the more progressive swingers. At that time you could buy them in metal tins, 12 to a tin, for $2.45 a box.
>
> Poppers, and their popularity, were the precursors to other drugs that quickly came on the scene. This usually started with grass which was smoked by almost everyone at gay cocktail parties. One was considered an outcast if he had a party and refused to allow grass to be smoked

on the deck of his apartment.

Shortly after the wide acceptance of grass we had the use of hash and its many derivatives, Thai stick ,etc. This gave an even more intense high, and the only disadvantage to this was the higher cost.

It was a short step to move to stronger chemicals. From this point on, the sky was the limit, and the limit was set by the individual based on his particular feelings about different drugs.

Drugs were used in the gay community solely to intensify the sexual experience. Drugs were used by gays regularly on the weekend, so the phones were very busy on Thursday and Friday evenings lining up the party favors for the weekend.

Most people experimented with acid in order to explore their minds, but usually came away with bad hangovers and had to have massive doses of Thorazine to "come down."

As a group, gays were never very big in heroin, and I believe that if we had an accurate census today, we would find very few heroin addicts that are gay. It is interesting to note also that cocaine never caught on in the gay community the way it did in the straight community.

Speed became the drug of choice for the gay community, and San Francisco by the late 70s had gained the reputation of being the speed capital of the world. Large numbers of gay people had a natural antipathy for needles, so "homemade" speed became the popular drug. This way, one could snort the drug, mix it with a drink and drink it, put it in tissue paper and swallow it or insert it into the rectal area, or dissolve it in water and use it intravenously. It was plentiful, cheap, and one could stay high for 24 hours at a cost of $25.

This white powder was popular among the gay population, the majority of whom snorted the drug through straws. This gave an immediate and euphoric "high" very similar to "poppers," but unlike "poppers," which lasted only about 5-10 minutes with the high, the speed would keep a person going all night. A person on speed had no trouble maintaining a perpetual erection.

Young people were able to engage all night in sex with large numbers of different individuals without the problem of orgasm, which was inhibited by the use of speed. This became a recreation addiction. While there was no physical withdrawal, the "high" was so pleasurable that most people found it difficult to stop.

The ultimate trip for drug users is called a "speed ball," which was a mixture of heroin and either speed or cocaine. The resultant "high" produced a very intense "rush" followed by enough mind alteration that a person was game for anything the mind could comprehend doing sexually.

Without the release of inhibition, the sexual aberrations would not have been possible, nor would the person have had the staying power to go all night. Most people immediately started having sex while they were "rushing," but some people preferred to get over the initial rush and then start having sex.

As a physician, of course I had known for years, as had all the doctors at San Francisco General, about our city's bathhouses. Although it was certainly "common" in San Francisco, I thought it was counterproductive to rich human bonding and terribly unhealthy physically. I saw it as a selfish lifestyle. It was hedonistic to the point of unbelievability, and, yes, I have to say that certain things I heard and saw were repugnant to me even then, long before we knew of AIDS.

But their lifestyle, when I became a doctor in the late sixties, was not part of my central concern. It was just something that was there. We had gay sex as we had crime and drugs and child abuse and many other manifestations of aberrant living, but I don't think I spent much time in thinking about it and bringing a value judgment to it. Even when I had to treat an enormous injury resulting from a bathhouse sexual incident, I would detach myself emotionally and see it as an injury that needed medical treatment.

There are many patients whom I routinely treat whose lifestyles are abhorrent to me—parents who abuse their children to the point of death, pimps who pour gasoline over their hookers and set them afire for having withheld their "pay"—that sort of thing. Over the years, I took care of many criminals from the San Quentin and Vacaville penitentiaries. I frequently treated the criminally insane. I have had to deal with worse lifestyles than those attributed to San Francisco's homosexuals.

Therefore, I trained myself as a physician to ignore what any homosexual patient might have done to bring about an injury. Regardless of the circumstances, I tried to do my best medically. I didn't pass judgment on them. I was just there as their doctor.

I don't remember when I took care of my first AIDS patient and I certainly do not remember any particular judgment I brought to his injurious lifestyle. My stance at that time was not a public health stance. As the saying goes, in literature as in love, one is at times astonished at what is chosen by others.

Let's say I was astonished.

That's how I felt in the beginning about the injuries I saw in numerous gay men. If and when they came to my hospital with an enormous injury from a specific practice in a bathhouse encounter, to me, it was just an injury. I was nobody's judge or jury; I simply fixed the injury.

But then the virus came.

These past few years, there have been some pretty unorthodox guesses about the origin of HIV. Who is to say where it originated? At this point, nobody knows. No one can say with any certainty how such a terrible illness started. My guess might be as good as yours. My guess is a medical guess.

It is based on what we know about how viruses mutate and strengthen themselves in their evolutionary struggle, losing weak particles as they "move up" via "hosts" to the point where they "take on a life of their own."

There are many viruses around, and some are hardier than others.

We as doctors have been taking care of infections such as unusual pneumonias or tuberculosis for many years and have been able to observe certain patterns at close quarters. We take care of chemotherapy and radiation therapy patients, for example, and these cancer patients are exceptionally prone to getting unusual and often fatal diseases from bacteria and viruses that normally would not be harmful.

These infections are called opportunistic infections.

When we took care of patients with opportunistic infections in the past, there was never any need to take any special precautions, except for tuberculosis, because we were healthy, and the bacteria and viruses inside our dying patients were no threat to us. While these bacteria and viruses were very hard on weakened people, they did not hurt the healthy.

When these patients died, their diseases died with them. That was the end of it.

It is quite possible, I think, that the AIDS virus was around for many years, but it may have been a harmless virus. I believe the first AIDS case has now been shown to have occurred as long ago as 1959. It did not attack the general population because it may not have been virulent enough.

But then, in the late 1960s and early 1970s, we saw the start of the Gay Revolution. That's when "love-ins" became the vogue; orgies might be a better word.

With it came practices in gay bathhouses with hundreds or even thousands of sexual partners per year engaged in all sorts of traumatic sex—promiscuous, abusive and violent sex, brutal, vicious and ramming sex that often involved tearing of the lining of the intestines and rectum so that there was direct contact with semen and blood between numerous partners in rapid succession.

Bathhouse is a misnomer. The only function of these establishments is to provide a place for non-stop anonymous sex of any type imaginable with as many partners as one wished.

As Mark described it recently:

When I came to San Francisco in 1961, the following gay bathhouses were in existence: Jack's on Post Street, The Club on Turk Street, Dave's on Washington (later moved to 100 Broadway) and the San Francisco Baths on Ellis opposite the side of the Hilton. All of these places catered to the gay crowd. All had steam rooms. Some had "hot rooms," and S.F. Baths had a pool.

By 1975 all of the above bathhouses were still in operation. In addition, we had 21st Street Baths located on 21st Street between Mission and Valencia, Ritch Street located on Ritch Street, The Barracks off Folsom Street, the Slot Hotel on Folsom at 6th, The Handball Express (which also went by several other names) located on Harrison at 6th, The Club on the corner of 8th and Folsom (now the Episcopal Sanctuary for the Homeless). The former Club Baths on Turk Street had been renamed but was still there. There was also Sutro Baths located at the corner of Folsom and 6th which was mainly homosexual but billed itself as being bisexual. On the weekends, there were women as well as men there.

The last two bathhouses to open were The Hothouse and Animals. Neither had a steam room, nor was there any interest in them being anything other than sex pleasure houses where one rented rooms, usually the size of a sleaze hotel room.

Some rooms were equipped with exotic equipment such as stockades, sling harnesses, mirrors, shackles etc. There was much fisting, group sex, exhibitionism and voyeurism. Again, each place seemed to have its own clientele and type of crowd. The younger crowd would go to The Baths at 8th and Howard while the raunchy leather crowd would go to either The Barracks, Animals or the Slot. You could purchase a variety of drugs there for intravenous or oral use if you knew the right person.

Physical contact at the bathhouses was made by the

usual method of eye contact, going into someone's room and shutting the door, having someone invite you into their room, grabbing someone in the halls and groping to determine penis size for those people where that was a number one priority.

In the "baths" there were also lockers, for there were never enough rooms to go around on the weekends, and some people used lockers because they were much cheaper. Then they cruised the halls with a towel around their waist, or in the kinky places with a variety of leather gear, with leather jockstraps, etc. The dress was limited only by one's imagination.

All had showers where a hose was hooked up. There was a diverter that changed water from going through the shower head to going through a long plastic hose which had been smoothed out on one end. This was inserted repeatedly into the rectum to clean out. Some people would spend literally hours doing this, almost getting off on that part of the preparation.

Here was a fairly self-contained population who appeared to be quite well as far as their overall health was concerned, but because of their sexual practices, virtually all had hepatitis or had had hepatitis.

They virtually all had venereal diseases or had had venereal diseases and had thereby weakened certain mucous tissues.

Many gays had intestinal parasites because of their back-and-forth fecal contamination from fisting and anal sex.

A large number of them were either on recreational drugs or hard drugs which heightened their need for sex and more sex and did away with all inhibitions.

Many had sex with multiple partners through "glory holes"—3-5 inch holes cut in the wall for the purpose of repeated, anonymous sex where participants never saw each other.

Here is Mark's description,

> One of the most obscene things I ever witnessed was in the late 70s at a bathhouse called The Barracks. The Barracks and the Slot and Animal were bathhouses that didn't bother having steam rooms, etc. They were more properly just sex hotels equipped for what their customers needed to have in the way of equipment to complete their fantasy trips.

> I noticed a young man cruising the halls of the Barracks. He had only a towel fastened around his waist. He had taken a hypodermic needle and filled it with about 40 units of an almost clear liquid which I assume was speed. He had tucked the needle behind his ear, in the manner that some men carry an extra cigarette. He was ready to go.

Here was a predator in search of prey.

Here was a milieu, with no hygienic considerations, where you could take a virus that really wasn't very virulent at first and pass it back and forth repeatedly and violently by means of blood and semen. Recalls Mark:

> Every perversion imaginable was done in the gay community. One can say that one experienced debauchery

similar to the days of Rome. The only difference was that the "slaves" were not for real, but could in some cases be just as abused.

There was no lack of bodies. There was no lack of bodily fluid exchange.

The virus was passed back and forth repeatedly among this very homogeneous population with certain medical characteristics and sex-specific tissue weaknesses. This gay bathhouse population comprised the walking wounded. They appeared healthy, but had numerous medical problems as outlined. Yet they were generally healthier than the group of patients initially prone to opportunistic infections, chemotherapy patients.

So what does a struggling virus or bacteria do when it starts climbing up the evolutionary ladder?

It starts getting stronger. And stronger and stronger.

Weak particles die off. A virus such as HIV is particularly prone to rapid mutation, sometimes within the same body.

That means that it can more easily infect progressively healthier people. These people then can infect still healthier people. That is one way a harmless virus can become a deadly virus. The rest may be called history.

Chronologically, this theory makes a lot of sense to many knowledgeable doctors. Since we now know that the incubation period between infection and manifestation of the disease can be as long as a decade, it may not be coincidence that in 1981 some ten years after "Gay Liberation" occurred we saw our first gay patients coming down with a disease that didn't even have a name.

It is common knowledge by now that at the outset, AIDS in America was an almost exclusively homosexual disease, appearing in cities such as New York, Los Angeles and San Francisco, cities with large gay populations. In fact, that was its initial name: GRIDS, Gay Related Immune Deficiency Syndrome.

It was in the bathhouses long before it was found in the streets. Drugs, prostitution, blood transfusions and bisexuality provided handy bridges to let it cross sex-preference boundaries.

Nature could have done it.

But anal sex specifically—and rampant promiscuity generally—helped.

Gay males have always been inordinately vulnerable to a host of infectious diseases, diseases often occurring simultaneously. Medically speaking, anal sex with multiple partners in rapid succession is not an innocuous practice. When Andy Rooney said that the homosexual lifestyle was unhealthy, he was medically correct. He was suspended from his job for telling the truth.

In medical circles, we speak of the "gay bowel syndrome" a descriptive term that refers to such unpretty things as intestinal pathogens and chronic infections.

Almost all gay males have or have had hepatitis B. Many gay males have ulcers and oozing blisters in or around the intestinal tracts, including the mouth and rectum.

More than half of all reported cases of syphilis in the United States occur in homosexual men.

Genital herpes is very common, as are anal warts.

Exchange of body fluids into these open sores and recurring lesions will irritate and compromise the mechanisms that make for a healthy immune system. The result is improper functioning of the immune system. The ability to fight infection is decreased.

There are physical injuries, too.

Nature simply has not equipped the tissue of the rectum for heavy-duty assault. Intestinal tissues bruise and tear easily during violent homosexual intercourse. The bowel will react with spasms. A tearing of the lining can occur, as well as bleeding anal fissures, small cracks in the anus when it is torn.

Brutal anal sex, "fisting," or the use of mechanical sexual aids such as dildos or vibrators produce tears and lacerations of the rectum throughout which infected semen and pathogenic organisms can and will enter the bloodstream. Blood and fecal matter sometimes find their way into the abdominal cavity through injuries.

Colitis, a severe inflammation of the mucous membrane of the colon, is not uncommon among gays.

Infected semen received into the mouth can also infect a partner through abrasions or lesions on the gums, tongue and roof of the mouth or even through intact mucosa.

In sum and summary, the picture of gay promiscuity, seen from a strictly medical point of view, is an invitation for disaster. As doctors, we see prolonged and repeated physical abuse and resulting trauma to very vulnerable body parts. We see injuries that have been piled on injuries. We see a lifestyle where hygiene is nil, thanks to shared bathhouse hose nozzles and feces. Urine and semen flow on to the floor and on to each other.

Medically speaking, the injuries are freakish. They are not injuries that we would routinely find in the heterosexual population or in the lesbian population.

Nature said "exit," not "enter," yet the things that have entered the exit are items that we as doctors have had to remove from the rectums of gay men: light bulbs, vegetables such as zucchinis and cucumbers that have already started fermenting, Coke bottles, dildos, vibrators, shaving cream cans.

I saw an X-ray once of a 3 inch by 12-inch plastic tool box before it had been removed from a homosexual's rectum—the tools were still inside.

I know of one case where plaster of Paris was used. It made for anxious moments in the operating room. The hardened stuff had to be removed in chips.

Patients have come into our hospitals who have sustained enormous injuries from violent, sadistic sex. Not infrequently, large foreign objects have punctured the intestinal wall, causing dangerous seepage of fecal matter into the abdomen.

Mark remembers a specific case:

Many gay people wanted other people to kill them in a trip. I met a guy once who wanted to be castrated because as a child he grew up on a farm and worshipped a man whose job it was to castrate the pigs on the farm.

My friend was about 13 or 14 when he developed this fascination for this man. He felt that way all of his life. He also wanted to be strangled to death and achieve orgasm at the moment of death.

He may have achieved his wish as he allowed someone high on speed to go with him to his house where the "speeder" handcuffed my friend to the bed and then strangled him to death.

The speeder stole many articles from my friend's house and then set the house on fire. This was in April of 1984. The man who committed the murder was apprehended, imprisoned in the Vacaville, California Penitentiary and recently has been released on parole.

While this may be an extreme example of sadomasochistic sex, an activity called "fisting" is not. Fisting is a common practice in the gay community.

It does just what it says: it's manual-anal intercourse.

One man will push his hand, fist and forearm up to his elbow into the rectum and lower colon of another man and sometimes grip and tear on the liver, spleen and intestinal wall.

Explained Mark:

> Fisting was accomplished by liberal use of Crisco with a person covering both hands and arms up to the elbows. Many men were able to be fisted up to the elbows with one hand and arm.

> There was a short homosexual who used to frequent The Slot who was very popular because he had no hands, his arms terminating above the wrist with rounded stumps. He was very popular with those into fisting.

In some cases, well documented in hospital records, the damage to the rectal sphincter from fisting is so extensive that a colostomy must be performed.

If fisting happens over an extended period of time, the rectal sphincter gets stretched. Not a few gay males have serious problems with rectal incontinence.

"Golden showers" are another well-known homosexual practice where some men will urinate on eager partners. Urination into the mouth and over the body of a participant, known inventively as "water sports," is a common homosexual practice.

Some homosexual males are known to have defecated on each other, a "sexual variation" known as scatting.

These practices are not part of an "acceptable alternate lifestyle" in a respectable medical book. Medically speaking, the homosexual lifestyle is a harmful lifestyle fueled by a sexual addiction that has no limits, knows no rules, and refuses to practice restraint.

And all this didn't happen yesterday. It is still going on. Here are remarks made by another homosexual:

> "Recently, these (homosexual) parties have become immensely popular, drawing considerably over a hundred people. . . ."

Eight years after the onset of AIDS and four years after the closing of the commercial baths, the once notorious San Francisco sex scene is obviously still flourishing.

Attitudes are cavalier at best. Is it dangerous? Not really, is the attitude. "It depends on the condition of my mouth," says one. "The virus is really fragile," says another.

There is a general sense that the epidemic is no longer as mysterious or pervasive as it once was.

"Gay men understand the situation much better now," explained Jim, a business consultant in his mid-thirties, at the East Bay event. "We're extremely well educated about the virus and how it is spread. Four or five years ago everything was suspect and people were in a panic syndrome. Some people are still paranoid, but it's not necessary as long as you exercise a little self-control and follow some limits."

Here is an excerpt of a recent write-up by Dawn Garcia in the San Francisco Chronicle:

> Five years after the city closed 14 gay bath houses and clubs to halt high-risk sexual activity, private clubs offering sex are thriving in San Francisco.
>
> The clubs, mostly converted apartments and back rooms of porno-video arcades and bookstores, are advertised weekly in the personal sections of the city's gay newspapers. Joining them is a simple matter of paying an admission fee of $1.
>
> "I was there on a Thursday afternoon, and there were 50 or 60 people there—it was like something out of the pre-AIDS era," said an AIDS patient who went to a South-of-Market club on Clementina Street and asked not to be named. . . .
>
> No current laws regulate such clubs. The city's closure of bathhouses in 1984 was limited to specific businesses named in a civil suit.
>
> Although health department officials acknowledged yesterday that risky sex without condoms may be going on again in private clubs in San Francisco, they said it did not appear to be a sizeable problem.
>
> "It's true that there is a tiny, tiny portion of people for whom high-risk sexual behavior is still a pastime," said Tom Peters, associate director of the San Francisco Department of Public Health. "I can't honestly say we're monitoring places, but we're having some policy discussions now about what action we should take". . . .
>
> There seemed to be no shortage of business at two South-of-Market clubs visited by a *Chronicle* reporter last week.

The Clementina Street club and another on Tehama Street are both advertised on a "Glory Hole Hotline," a telephone recording that lists the clubs' hours of operations and events. ...

On one visit by a reporter, about 40 men were there, watching X-rated videos in a living room area, buying beer or sodas from the kitchen and engaging in oral and manual sex.

© San Francisco Chronicle
Reprinted by permission.

Lise Von Susteren, a psychiatrist in private practice in Washington, D. C., in a write-up for *This World,* described the lethal attitude of one of her AIDS patients:

Full of dread, I asked him if he was now having sex with anyone.

Yes, he was.

Was he using condoms or taking other protective steps?

No—except when people asked, which was rare.

I couldn't believe it. Did he know that the AIDS virus would likely kill everyone who had it?

Yes, sort of.

Did he realize that having sex with people was almost like handing them a death sentence?

He guessed so.

A gay weekly newspaper in San Francisco had this to say in a write-up entitled *Late Eighties Sex Scene: Safety and Variety.*

The other so-called San Francisco sex clubs, the porno bookstores, also survived the closures (of the bathhouses).

Cruising and sex have, of course, always taken place in such places, but the activities seem to have intensified in the past few years. Two bookstores, one on Polk and one on Folsom, are particularly popular, each possessing its expert regulars.

"There are rhythms and flows to the crowd," explains Tom, a good-looking, lean and muscular man in his mid-thirties, who stops by the Polk bookstore often. "Certain days and hours are better than others. Mondays, for example, are suprisingly good, and, of course, lunch and after work are always busy with at least 25 people."

Like the bath houses of old, the porno bookstores are especially useful in obtaining non-disruptive sex outside of a relationship. Tom, who has lived in San Francisco for fifteen years and has had a lover for the last ten, has a number of ongoing involvements at the bookstores.

"I've been having sex with the same people for years at the bookstore," he confides. "We know exactly what the other likes sexually, though otherwise we barely know each other. My lover knows all about this, and doesn't mind as long as I come home every night. You might not believe this but, except for travel reasons, we've never spent a night away from each other."

Interestingly, this is what the homosexual community calls a long-term "stable" relationship.

There is no escaping the evidence that gay-specific practices have fueled HIV in the United States. The evidence is overwhelming that the vast majority of hemophiliacs and other blood recipients have fallen prey to AIDS infection as a direct consequence of blood donated by homosexuals with the AIDS virus, whether knowingly infected or not.

The evidence is in the numbers and in the geography.

A few years ago, the ratio of male to female AIDS cases was 14 to 1, and while the gap has narrowed, more males than females continue to be stricken by the disease, and most of those victims are gays.

It is estimated that today three out of four AIDS-stricken people on the American continent are male homosexuals. In New York and San Francisco, 70 percent of male homosexuals are estimated to be infected with the AIDS virus and are infectious to others. There is no avoiding the evidence; it is on the map and in the numbers. AIDS exploded in the bathhouses frequented by homosexuals.

It was passed back and forth by homosexuals in bushes, public restrooms, porno shops and adult bookstores. It is still spreading there by much-unaltered practices. It spreads as if there were no tomorrow, as indeed, there may not be.

While for a time it seemed as though the homosexual community had learned to practice more restraint in the wake of massive initial infections, the evidence now seems to indicate that nothing much has changed.

The deadly virus, sad to say, has made little difference in sexual practices in the homosexual community. AIDS spreads because, as in the past, so now, gay male sex is still the old variety: sadistic, masochistic, promiscuous, hedonistic, contemptuous, anonymous, and unhygienic in the extreme. I see the results in the Emergency Room.

The "decrease" in additional numbers of gays becoming infected, a "fact" so often referred to in media coast-to-coast, is a spurious one: if most gays are already infected, there will be "fewer" new infections.

Many gays themselves will say that there is something profoundly cold and contemptuous in many homosexual practices. Take a look at these ads, published a few months ago:

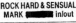

This matters from a medical perspective because it makes for promiscuous sex without the possibility of contact-tracing. How can our health care system warn potentially infected sexual partners of danger and urge sexual responsibility when partners number in the hundreds and "love" is made through a hole in the wall with not a single word exchanged?

Kirk and Madsen address promiscuous homosexuality at length:

> First and foremost is the peculiarly shallow way in which gay men tend to select their associates. . . .One passes, in effect, all candidates for personal attention through the sieve of sexual attraction.
>
> The practice of repeatedly going to bed with men about whom one knows, and cares, nothing, tends eventually to harden into a habitual shallowness, and a disinclination to judge by more important criteria.
>
> The magic code word which we've all heard until we could puke, is hassles. What Joe Gay is looking for, he'll tell you, is a "hassle-free" relationship, in which his lover isn't "overinvolved," "doesn't make demands," and "gives him enough space." In reality, no amount of space could ever be enough, because what Joe is really looking for isn't a lover at all, but a handsome. . . sort of low-maintenance household appliance.

The authors aptly summarize the situation, "Gay men can feel free to treat unsatisfactory relationships like Kleenex: one blow and out you go!"

Readers shocked with the above will probably remember that a passionate case has often been made by people sympathetic to the homosexual lifestyle, which is that many homosexual unions are close emotional unions that last over a very long period of time.

It is possible these individuals exist.

There may be gay men out there who act as mature and responsible people. They probably try to practice "safe sex," although sex even with condoms is not safe sex. We can assume they form meaningful and nourishing relationships, sustain each other emotionally and protect each other physically. Should AIDS befall them, they keep to themselves, comfort each other and do not step out on the town to find an uninfected partner for relief.

That is the ideal, and many people vouch that such relationships exist.

However, a very large number of gay men are interested only in one night stands with multiple anonymous partners. Many homosexual men privately admit that there is no permanent bonding in their relationships. Sure, two men may live together for long periods of time but that doesn't mean that they have a lasting, intimate, caring relationship. They may stay together for financial reasons or for convenience, but the caring part of the relationship ends soon and one or both are out pursuing as much anonymous sex as they can find.

These are the ones I am talking about, these who have for years and years, compromised their health, their partners' health, their community's health and now their country's health by their bizarre sexual conduct and promiscuous sexual practices.

I want to go on record saying strongly that I have now revised my tolerance scales. I do bring judgment to male homosexual behavior. I do so as a physician and I do so as a citizen.

When certain sexual practices and preferences are killing not just the practitioners, but also scores of innocent people who have nothing to do with that lifestyle—didn't choose it, don't endorse it but on the other hand, have never harmed it either—is it not right to speak up loudly and be heard?

The gay male consumption in terms of random partners has been overwhelming. We are talking numbers. We are talking death. We are talking promiscuity on a scale that is hard to fathom, and that has to stop.

A good place to start would be to shut down the bathhouses, (yes, many are still open) and the porno-video shops—now! In addition to the city parks and public restrooms, these are the places where much of the random, anonymous sex takes place. Why don't the militant gay-rights activists shut them down?

Specifically, where is ACT-UP to help us?

A fine and sure-fire way to gain respect, cooperation and compassion within the heterosexual community for the appalling homosexual plight would be to do just that.

Responsible gay men know this and a few are beginning to speak out against gay promiscuity, as do Kirk and Madsen when they write: "What can we say of a man who places his desire to continue to have orgasms ahead of his partner's desire to continue to live?" They speak of Gaetan Dugas, the airline steward, who early in the epidemic had sex with hundreds of men in the bathhouses, then turned up the lights and proclaimed, "I have gay cancer and I will die. Now you will die, too."

Kirk and Madsen continue: "While Dugas's case is extreme, the tendency illustrated is by no means isolated. Rock Hudson's biographies indicate a similar pattern of self-deception leading—potentially fatally—to the deception of others."

And, finally, let's put to rest the argument that homosexuals can't change. That is an old, old argument—and in the trash it goes. "No doubt," said A. A. Milne, "Jack the Ripper excused himself on the grounds that it was human nature." Human nature, above all, consists in understanding and applying moral mandates. Maybe homosexuals can't change the object of their sexual attraction, but they don't have to act on their impulses, especially when it can kill themselves or others.

I say that a medical judgment that strengthens a moral mandate demands subsequent curbs on behavior. This is now more appropriate than ever.

But sadly, the strength of such judgment, or lack thereof, may well be a function of AIDSpeak.

We must alter our language. This truth must be repeated, over and over again: Somebody's private mania is spreading massive public death.

The independent variable that has changed the liberal tolerance equation and has the power to alter the globe, is a virus.

In these perilous times, being a homosexual or bisexual does not any longer mean, as it did in the Happy Sixties Salad Days, that these experimental sexual antics can safely be part of your garden variety barbeque set.

Say Kirk and Madsen:

> Straights hate gays not just for what their myths and lies say we are, but also for what we really are. In one major aspect, America's homohaters have, like the proverbial blind pig, rooted up the truffle of truth: the gay lifestyle—not our sexuality, but our lifestyle—is the pits.

Creeps misbehave because it gets them what they want. They will not cease to misbehave until misbehavior ceases to be worth their while. Since the laws cannot punish lower-order misbehavior, it is left up to the victim and the bystander to mete out punishment. The only form of punishment available to private citizens, yet not intolerably disruptive, is social censure.

So speak up! Instead of privately deploring the cheap antics you see going on around you, put your popularity on the line, and speak up for what you believe. It's as simple as that.

They are right. AIDS was simply not part of the original script.

Since we have only one small planet and don't want civil war, perhaps now is the time for the homosexual community to be as diligent in pursuit of their responsibilities as they are in pursuit of their rights.

This point is summarized quite beautifully in this short paragraph with which the authors close their book, and with which I'd like to close my chapter:

For twenty immature years, the gay community has shrieked for rights while demonstrating an alarming degree of irresponsibility. If gays expect straights ever to accord them their rights, this is one of the things that must change. We must cease to be our own worst enemies.

6

The Old Party Line

As though it were the Gospel, we hear that HIV does not transmit through household contact, animal vectors, such as cats, cows or sheep or insect bites.

It does not, we are told, transmit by air.

You can't get HIV, says AIDSpeak, through hugging and kissing.

You can't get it if somebody, AIDS-infected and near death, sneezes or coughs next to you. No way can you or anybody get it, the finger-shaking zealot tells you, from a handshake, a door knob, or a public restroom toilet seat.

The louder we shout, the more we will frighten the virus?

Please note this carefully: I am not saying here, nor have I ever said, that widespread AIDS transmission via household contact, animals or insects is a fact.

I am saying, I don't know. Our so-called "experts" don't know either, even though they say they do. The investigation has not been done.

The statistics I have seen that point toward the

possibility of non-acknowledged transmission are frightening. It is no longer warranted to warn against "high-risk behaviors" only, because "low-risk" populations now get AIDS, too.

Authorities, in order to keep people calm, have taken advantage of correlational studies and assigned "high risk" categories to infected people who may have contracted AIDS by innocuous means.

Let me explain.

If you look out of your window and you notice your sidewalk is wet, you cannot categorically conclude that it is wet because it rained.

Chances are that it *was* rain. It could have been rain. It could also have come from your sprinkler.

It could have been both.

It could have gotten wet from your sprinkler *before* it got wet from the rain.

If you see someone with AIDS, it could have been from anal sex with someone who had AIDS, but could it have been from sharing a toothbrush, a utensil or a kiss with someone who had AIDS? Most sexually involved people will *also* have casual contact.

It is true that there is a high correlation between "high risk" behavior and AIDS. It is also true that there is a high correlation between red hair and freckles. Red hair does not "cause" freckles, however, nor do freckles "cause" red hair. An underlying factor causes both.

Just because there is a strong correlation between high risk behavior and the incidence of AIDS, it does not warrant the intellectual quantum leap that other forms of transmission can be categorically ruled out.

We can't afford to guess. We must study the causative factors, for underestimating this disease statistically by studies only in high risk populations may spell doom for hundreds of thousands of victims whom authorities believe to be at "low risk."

We must know precisely. In order to know, we must look.

Ringing and unfounded claims regarding AIDS in low-risk populations are made via epidemiological studies and not via basic research. Let me explain.

These epidemiological studies are, in essence, of two kinds: those that compare groups with each other at a fixed point in time and those that follow one group over a period of time. The first are called cross-sectional studies. The second are called longitudinal studies.

Vastly simplified, a cross-sectional study compares, let's say, the insect damage to peaches during the month of June.

It says nothing of peaches infected by insects in May, July or any other month.

We can't extrapolate beyond our peaches studied during June.

If we want to answer certain questions over time, we would design a longitudinal study.

If we were to answer questions, let us say, about insect damage to our peaches during their growth and ripening, we would take repeated measurements from the same peach trees during certain intervals.

If we want to have a comprehensive picture of the insect damage, we would take repeated measurements until there was no doubt left whatsoever about what insects do to peaches.

If we take our measurements through June, July, or August, find that the damage that we see is minimal, and then forecast that there's no way the insect will cause damage in

September, what happens if September rolls around? Our beetles love our peaches in September!

Similarly, cross-sectional studies that try to answer certain questions about AIDS are very limited in scope and answer only part of what we really want to know.

For instance, if we compare the count of new infections in households with AIDS compared to households without AIDS, we can't infer that just because there is no AIDS today in either home from household contact, there won't be infections tomorrow.

Our count is the count for today.

If we decide to do our counting over time, we must count long enough. The count should be at least three-and-a-half years, at present our best estimate for the maximum time required for antibodies to develop to the AIDS virus.

Most longitudinal studies have been short-term and have been abandoned too early. They evaluated the households for only a year, while some were as short as three months. Let's start with what is called household transmission. The final word on household transmission has not yet been spoken.

When I talked to Dr. James Curran of the Centers for Disease Control about a year ago, I asked if any substantive household contact studies were still being conducted.

"No, they have all been discontinued," replied Dr. Curran.

Out of Russia, meanwhile, comes word that transfusion-infected babies have given AIDS to their mothers.

The Child Welfare League has said that as many as 30,000 children and youths in the United States will be HIV-positive by 1991. Many of them will need homes when their parents die of HIV-related causes.

A thought-provoking article suggests at least the possibility of insects as vectors of infection. I quote here from a 1989 publication in *Archives of Dermatology*[1], commenting on skin lesions observed in AIDS patients.

> "these pruritic (itching) skin lesions were an initial symptom in 79% of patients. They were the first and only initial sign and symptom of AIDS in 45% of the patients...
>
> Initially the lesions resembled insect bites and many patients assumed they were secondary to mosquitoes...
>
> The apparent geographic restriction of these pruritic eruptions to tropical areas suggests an environmental factor such as insects or an allergic phenomenon...
>
> There was no association between these pruritic eruptions and any particular opportunistic infections that would suggest that they were a cutaneous (skin) manifestation of the systemic infection. Finally, we must also consider whether the pruritic skin lesions might be a consequence of primary human immunodeficiency virus infection of the skin."

The AIDS virus in man is *strikingly similar* to the AIDS-like virus found in animals, and some of these animal viruses do transmit readily from one animal to another through casual contact or via aerosols or sprays that are created by coughing or sneezing.

We must keep an open mind. We need respectable scientific evidence to verify or to refute transmission routes not presently acknowledged. We must not mix our messages so that the evidence, if troubling, does not get watered down by wishful thinking, human rights rhetoric, car bumper stickers or T-shirt slogans.

Consider this article, an unholy mixture of serious science and AIDSpeak. It is entitled "Cats and AIDS" and appeared in July of 1990 in *Discover*.

The strange illness first surfaced in three cats in California, shortly after AIDS began spreading in the human population in the early eighties. A distraught cat lover had brought her ailing pets to Niels Pedersen, a professor of veterinary medicine at the University of California at Davis, on a prophetic hunch that the animals were suffering from an AIDS-like disease. The cats, which later died, were plagued by a host of opportunistic diseases, including respiratory infections and lesions of the mouth and skin.

Studies have since revealed that the cats were indeed infected by a virus that has much in common with the human AIDS virus. Feline Immunodeficiency Virus, or FIV, kills T cells and gradually causes the collapse of the animal's immune system. And under the microscope FIV and its human counterpart look eerily alike.

Now the feline virus's genes have been decoded, making a more detailed comparison possible. The cat and human viruses are "cousins" on the retrovirus family tree, says John Elder, a molecular biologist at the research foundation of Scripps Clinic in La Jolla, who collaborated with Pedersen in the study. But, ironically, the evidence from stored blood samples suggests that the cat virus was around long before the human one arrived in this country. "The virus was always there," says

Elder. "But it took the experience of the AIDS virus to bring it to light."

One striking difference is that cats transmit the virus mainly through bites. "A cat's tooth penetrates the skin much like a hypodermic needle, so transmission is very efficient," Pedersen explains. "One bite is enough to cause infection." (Fortunately, it's biologically impossible for cats to transmit their virus to humans.) Studies indicate that as many as 5 percent of the country's free-roaming felines—cats that spend a lot of time outdoors or strays—are infected. Now research is under way to find a treatment or, better still, a vaccine to protect the animals. Cats may yet turn out to be man's best friend. Their illness parallels the human one, says Elder, providing a natural AIDS model.

Why the coy qualification in parentheses? And why the Pollyanna conclusion?

We have been wrong before. We have erroneously concluded many times before that HIV transmission just couldn't happen in ways that we found troublesome.

Here is a capsule summary of how tragically and disastrously we have been wrong before.

At first, HIV was called "gay cancer" or GRID—Gay Related Immunodeficiency Disease. It seemed that it "preferred" a certain kind of homosexual, one who liked anal sex. It was a cancer, wasn't it?

Conclusion: Cancers did not transmit.

The cancer next identified as Kaposi's sarcoma was only part of the picture, we learned. There was serious immune suppression, but the mysterious illness still clustered around gay males.

Conclusion: It wouldn't jump gender to females.

Over time we did admit, because we had no other choice, that HIV was irrefutably, a sexually transmitted disease. It struck both males and females.

Conclusion: No way did it transmit non-sexually.

The most respected researchers in the United States believed for quite some time that sexual transmission, primarily anal sex, was now the one and only way the virus would transmit.

When people started casting jaundiced eyes in the direction of the blood banks, their fears were ridiculed.

No way, the zealots said.

Doctors questioning the safety of the blood banks ran into enormous skepticism and, often, caustic ridicule.

America learned next that not only did the blood banks help spread the disease, they spread it with AIDSpeak that rang from the mountains. Even after it was known that AIDS would spread that way, it was denied. This was unfortunate for patients who had had transfusions; to have haplessly received bad blood in a legitimate and medically sanctioned way turned out to be as deadly as a vial of cyanide, not just for them, but for their partners and, sadly, for 40 percent of the children delivered from an infected mother.

Still, we clutched onto what we now "knew" was "certainty," that women with non-transfused heterosexual partners couldn't contract HIV. It was still "clearly and demonstrably" a gay male disease that had found its way "by accident" into the general blood supply.

Some women became HIV-positive.

But only prostitutes, right? Maybe addicts. The virus was

still seen as a remarkably discriminating virus that could tell clean folks from the sleazies.

Slowly but surely, we learned some additional facts: this virus respected no demographics, no bank accounts, no age and no college degree. It transmitted to women and children. It transmitted to very old people, as well as to infants not yet in their cribs.

It transmitted to Ray Cohn and Rock Hudson. It transmitted in Hollywood, and it transmitted in Billings, Montana.

I remember all that vividly. The news has become progressively worse.

It seems that it was only yesterday when we were told that there was not even the remotest danger in occupational exposure such as through needlesticks. I have no patience whatsoever now with so-called "experts" when they tell me today that I can't be infected by being in contact with HIV-positive patients through body fluids other than blood.

Unless I see scientific proof convincing me beyond a shadow of a doubt that casual contact just cannot happen, I will reserve the right to say, "Show me that I am wrong in ways I can respect."

AIDSpeak has conditioned us not to shout, "Fire!"

There is a roaring fire, but if we just keep from acknowledging fire, then maybe it will self-destruct. With credits to Saul Bellow, a great deal of intelligence can be invested in ignorance when the need for illusion is deep.

I happen to believe that shouting, "Fire!" is appropriate. Had we done that twelve years ago, we would not now have 83,000 dead and 1 to 3 million Americans infected.

In 1980 it was believed that AIDS did not transmit at all.

In 1981 it was believed that AIDS did not transmit through blood transfusions. It took 14,000-16,000 victims with HIV from transfusions to get our authorities to admit that death was being kept refrigerated and frozen in blood bank inventories and that, maybe, it was time to test.

In 1983 it was believed that AIDS did not transmit heterosexually—at least not in America. In Africa, maybe—but surely not here!

In 1987 it was believed that needlesticks were harmless.

We now believe, in 1991, as if this wisdom has come down to us in stone slabs from Mount Sinai, that HIV does not transmit to children living in a household where there is HIV.

The general public stance is that this virus can't transmit via kissing, through sharing of utensils, by shaking hands or via aerosols. One risks professional lynching, practically, if one suggests mosquitoes, bedbugs, ticks or flies.

These claims of non-transmission are being made because there is no clear-cut "evidence" that HIV transmits that way. The truth is no one has done the proper studies. As things stand now, authorities claim they don't know of any AIDS in American children who live in households that have HIV or go to school with children who are HIV-infected, even though scientific evidence now tells us clearly that *it may take ten years or longer to develop the symptoms of AIDS.*

We haven't yet tested that many children or "low risk" adults, for that matter.

We *simply don't know* whether or not this virus transmits

through casual contact or other vectors, and if it transmits, to what degree.

We must start asking questions.

The Centers for Disease Control, the Surgeon General and all the public health authorities, coast to coast, toe the official party line, that AIDS can be transmitted only in four specific ways—"sex, sharing of needles, passed on from mother to newborn and from HIV-contaminated blood transfusions." They deny that AIDS can, may and probably is being transmitted in troubling additional ways.

One way that documented transmission happens is, of course, by sexual activity, primarily through homosexual sex which is predominantly anal sex, and additionally by regular heterosexual activity.

AIDS does transmit, as we now know, through the exchange of blood, saliva and semen via mucous membranes, both injured and intact. In addition, as I will show, it transmits through injured and through intact skin.

It is now recognized that transmission from mother to child can occur, not just prenatally through the placenta (as most lay people blithely believe) but at birth by coming in contact with HIV-positive blood (by swallowing or inhaling it), or after birth through mother's milk.

A few years ago we didn't think that that could happen, either.

We learned to our dismay that sharing of needles in seedy shooting galleries could easily transmit the lethal virus. We haven't yet absorbed the possibility that piercing your earlobes in an upper income shopping mall might transmit it just as easily.

We keep swallowing AIDSpeak—that is, the general notion that it is very difficult to "catch" the deadly virus.

It may be easier than we think. In fact, it may catch us.

It took a lot of casualties for the authorities to change their minds about the ways of transmission admitted above. Will we, a few years from now, be forced to make similar concessions regarding feces, urine, tears and other body fluids?

How many dead bodies does it take for us to start looking? Do we need a body count? Can we not reason from evidence presently known that casual transmission might happen?

Which puts the problem right up front.

What is casual transmission to you may not be the same definition authorities use.

Teacher-student contact is considered casual contact and is said not to be dangerous even if a student is infected. If that same teacher stops a nosebleed in an HIV-positive student, that would not be called casual contact any more. The teacher would be criticized for not using "universal precautions" to protect her hands from the infective blood, even though she has been told repeatedly that her working situation is free of risk.

In a hospital setting, it would clearly be called occupational transmission. Why is blood on a nurse's hand different from blood on a teacher's hand?

What begins as casual contact can suddenly change to "contact with another person's blood" in any situation where human beings interact.

That means there's no guarantee that what begins as casual contact will remain risk-free. To classify most working environments as only casual contact is unjustified and misleading because accidents involving blood have happened in every working situation.

If virus is present, then it may transmit.

We know it is present in almost all body fluids as well as blood. The prudent thing to do is to assume it will transmit through all body fluids.

With that hypothesis beneath our feet, the next scientific step would be to verify or to refute.

Are diapers dangerous?

Is it safe to let an AIDS-infected baby drool liberally on a shoulder?

And what about those toilet seats in San Francisco's airports?

When I ask these and other questions of my professional colleagues, I notice that they find it difficult to even grant my questions as legitimate, much less that my concern might be not only legitimate but crucial.

The chorus is: It cannot happen. It simply can't happen.

There is an almost criminal unwillingness to admit at least the possibility that *additional ways of transmission do exist, at least in theory, and are now being slowly documented in the literature as having actually occurred.*

Here's why.

We have a country that serves as a precedent of what can happen if this disease is left unchecked. In Zaire, one in three people now carries the virus. Among them are hundreds of thousands of children. There are no data on these children. Not all of them, we can deduce, have contracted the disease the only way we hope and pray and wish to believe it transmits.

There has been widespread and systematic government

indoctrination against a healthy fear of AIDS. If something is repeated long enough, it takes on a life of its own. It becomes a "self-evident" truth.

Said Anatole France, "If fifty million people hold a foolish notion, it is still a foolish notion."

Belief in itself, pro or con, is no proof of anything. For centuries it was believed the earth was flat and bigger than the sun. Within our lifetime it was held that man would never reach the moon.

A virus transmits if conditions are right.

If it is present in body fluids, other than blood, and we now *know* that it is present and active in tears, saliva, semen, breast milk, vaginal secretions, urine, cerebrospinal fluid and amniotic fluid, we must assume it *may* transmit that way.

We must start asking: When? How? Where? How often?

In fact, we have some evidence that it transmits not just in theory but in practice.

The documented evidence, at present, is in only a few cases:

* It transmits in saliva.[2,3]
* It transmits by blood-on-blood through open wounds.[4]
* There is evidence that it transmits through intact skin.[5]
* It will transmit after having been frozen.[6]
* It transmits through artificial insemination.[7]

What we don't know, at present, is the *degree* to which it transmits. We haven't really looked. We haven't really asked. Does it take a certain viral quantity before it will transmit? Does it take co-factors, such as a sufficiently weakened immune system?

This is not your garden-variety virus. This is a virus that takes its time, first in the ways it triggers antibodies, which may take as long as three and one half years, and then with developing symptoms, which may take as long as a decade. It is also a virus that likes to mutate rapidly, and we know that progressive mutations will make transmission more likely. We must take seriously the supposition that if conditions are right, this deadly virus will transmit. We must study the conditions under which it may transmit.

Said Dr. James Curran on "60 Minutes", refuting my claim that the virus may transmit through bloody aerosols in the operating room, "It's got to be done with facts."

Exactly. Where are his facts that bloody aerosols do not transmit?

Aerosols are tiny particles that remain airborne indefinitely. You breathe them into your lungs. Officials from the Centers for Disease Control have stated numerous times during television interviews that aerosols are not a problem. But, in print they say that aerosols *are* potentially dangerous.

> ...the CDC states:
> In the laboratory, the skin (especially when scratches, cuts, abrasions, dermatitis, or other lesions are present) and mucous membranes of the eye, nose, mouth, *and possibly the respiratory tract* should be considered as potential pathways for entry of virus.[8] (Italics added)

Even in the "60 Minutes" segment broadcast September 24, 1989, and re-broadcast August 5 of 1990, Dr. James Curran, head of HIV and AIDS for the Centers for Disease Control stated that there was no evidence that aerosols were dangerous.

You would assume that if he made that kind of a statement, he would have facts to back it up.

A colleague of mine wrote to the CDC and asked for all

of their information on HIV and aerosols. This was done under the Freedom of Information Act. The CDC officials wrote back that they have no information whatsoever on HIV and aerosols.

Can HIV transmit through airborne viral particles, particularly surgically created aerosols? It surely appears to be possible.

It started with my hunch that if the papilloma virus, a venereal wart virus, could become airborne via aerosols in the laser smoke plume, as had been documented in the medical literature[9] why not the AIDS virus also? During surgery, I drilled and reamed with power tools. I knew that there were bloody aerosols.

I knew, in addition, because I checked it out, that surgical masks would only filter out particles 5 microns or larger. I knew that the AIDS virus was 0.1 microns in size, many times smaller than a 5 micron particle. These viral particles, if airborne, could go through my surgical mask like BBs through a tennis net. Besides, no surgical masks have a tight fit—it would be easy for those lethal viral particles to " go around the rim."

We started investigating this possibility at the University of California and a laboratory team started looking at this problem simultaneously at Stanford University.

Dr. Greg Johnson, an orthopedic surgeon at Stanford, and Dr. William Robinson of the Infectious Disease Department did the following experiment:

They used a rotating drill bit which is like the drills we use on bone in the operating room. They dropped HIV-positive blood on the rotating drill bit while it was spinning rapidly.

Nine inches away, they put a 20 inch length of IV tubing, 2 millimeters in diameter. They put three coils in it so any blood that splattered around would settle on the walls of the tube.

The only air that would come out at the end of the tube, 20 inches away from the rotating drill bit, would be "clear" air.

That air was then bubbled through a culture of human mononuclear cells.

That air infected the cells with HIV .[10]

Let this sink in: the virus can stay alive and infective in the air 20 inches away from the rotating drill bit in what looks like clear air.

That is the distance from a surgeon's hand while he is working, to his mouth and nose. Live virus is being breathed in routinely during surgery.

Does it infect a surgeon if it infects the human lymphocytes in an experiment? Nobody seems to know.

This work has been expanded. Dr. Don Jewett has done work at the University of California on blood aerosolization during operating room procedures.

He has found that *blood from a patient sick with AIDS can infect a monkey and probably a human as well, in a quantity so small that the blood covers an area no bigger than the head of a pin.*

The mucous membranes of your nose and mouth are are packed with Langerhans cells. They can transport the virus[11] from the outside surface of the mucous membranes to the inside, as I will show with a subsequent study done by a respectable scientist abroad.

Here is part of the "60 Minutes" interview with Dr. James Curran of the Centers for Disease Control pertaining to potential aerosol danger:

Interviewer: One of the things (Dr. Day) thinks the CDC should be doing is to investigate the possible transmission of the virus through aerosols — a fine mist of blood and body fluids that occurs when surgeons cut into bone with drills and power saws. It's one of the reasons she wears her space suit. The CDC says there is no factual or theoretical basis for the transmission of the virus through aerosols, and places the chances at zero.

Curran: There's sometimes a fine line between evangelism and demagoguery. And the evangelists are important in order to change society. It's gotta be done with facts.

Interviewer: Is Dr. Day in your mind a demagogue or an evangelist?

Curran: I've never met her. The attributions would suggest a little of both.

I am pleased to report that, thanks to the pressure applied through that broadcast and elsewhere, the CDC has finally agreed to fund some studies on aerosols and possible transmission including the work we started at the University of California, San Francisco. But the change of heart by the CDC occurred only after I had challenged the authorities, been vilified for being "unscientific," and after 30 million people heard it stated twice on prime time documentary television across America and probably around the world that it was just evangelism and demagoguery to even consider the possibility that transmission might happen that way.

That's AIDSpeak.

If there is smoke, it is not "unscientific" to assume that, sooner or later, there will be a fire somewhere.

There is plenty of smoke at the present.

A nurse was overheard commenting recently: "We know a great deal already about that old virus." She saw herself as fully informed.

I'm sorry, but she's uninformed. The virus isn't "old." It's new in terms of our understanding and defenses. It is perplexing. There's much to learn. It would be beneficial to keep an open mind.

Unluckily, however, for our way of life, and our children's way of life (if there is any way of life left if we persist in our foolish course) we are doing so with a reluctance, timidity and lethargy as though we think we can swindle the virus.

We think that if we kind of trick it into leaving us alone as long as we leave it alone or shout our slogans loud enough about our human rights philosophy, then maybe it will vanish.

Transmission through non-sexual, non-blood pathways can happen, maybe not often, but often enough. It will be once too often for the one who becomes infected that way.

Let's start with what is known. Live virus has been found in blood, semen, breast milk, vaginal secretions, saliva, tears, urine, cerebrospinal fluid and amniotic fluid,"[12]   admits the

CDC.

Yet "universal precautions," according to the CDC, while now applying to all handling of blood and blood products, do not apply to sputum, tears and urine.[13,14]

The CDC states, furthermore, that transmission has not yet been documented by exposure to feces, nasal secretions, sweat, tears, urine and vomitus. Note that the argument is not that the virus cannot be found in those body fluids. *The argument is that transmission has not yet been proved.*

Why not?

According to one CDC release, experiments were set up to investigate transmission by body fluids, but "blood was found to transmit the disease most readily, so persons exposed to other body fluids subsequently were excluded from the study."[15]

I see.

If you eliminate from the study those people who have been exposed to other body fluids, you can be virtually certain that transmission by other body fluids will not be documented. How convenient!

There is an old saying: "Never let a fool kiss you, or a kiss fool you."

Wise words in light of the fact that the lethal virus has been not only detected in saliva, but has transmitted through saliva. It may come as a shock to the romantically inclined, but a few people seem to have contracted AIDS through kissing or saliva-on-skin exposure.

In April of 1990, I did a segment for a syndicated television show. The person introducing my appearance on this show teased the intended audience in a pre-broadcast ad by saying that I had a "shocking controversial claim." That shocking controversial claim was that there existed as of October, 1989, four reported cases of salivary transmission.

"Only four cases?" the skeptics will say. "Four cases after thirteen years?"

Yet in 1983, the CDC had documented only a few cases of AIDS transmission through blood transfusion. No doubt some people called that "shocking" in those years.

Now AIDS transmission via a blood transfusion is recognized as one of the three most common means of infection.

Two cases of saliva transmission are briefly summarized below:

A young boy age five in Germany died of AIDS from a blood transfusion, but before he died he gave AIDS to his 8-year old brother either through household contact (which is not supposed to occur), or through a bite witnessed by the mother *that did not break the skin.*[16]

A woman, age 72, contracted AIDS from a blood transfusion. She gave it to her husband, age 70, presumably through kissing because they had not had sex for many years.[17]

The health care authorities have been inconsistent even when they have admitted that transmission through saliva may exist. Here is one quirky mental acrobatic performed by health officials at the Centers for Disease Control pertaining to HIV known to be found in saliva.

The CDC has reasoned that it is unnecessary to follow "universal precautions" in regard to saliva exposure *except in the dental office.*[18]

What is it about dentistry that only dentists are at risk

regarding HIV found in saliva? Why not a nurse who handles sputum specimens in a hospital? Why not a nurse's aide who cleans up vomitus? Why not a postal worker who handles hundreds of letters with postage stamps that have been licked by postal customers?

AIDSpeak has been vociferous with regards to saliva as a means of potential infection. When Rock Hudson gave that kiss to Linda Evans only weeks before he died, America felt patriotically redeemed.

The former Surgeon General of the United States has stated categorically that AIDS cannot be transmitted by saliva.[19] According to present CDC guidelines, a nurse or technician handling sputum specimens is not even required to use gloves.

The American Heart Association, on the other hand, concerned about exposure via saliva, has issued its own guidelines allowing rescue workers performing cardiopulmonary resuscitation to avoid direct mouth-to-mouth contact with unconscious victims.[20]

It is impossible to reconcile these different health care standards regarding the perceived or real dangers of saliva. The issue at hand is not complex philosophically or costly to check out in practice.

Either saliva is potentially infectious or it is not.

It does not take a hundred documented cases to prove there is transmission. It does not even take five cases. It takes only one.

It took only one documented case of bone graft transmission of AIDS to get the CDC to write guidelines regarding frozen donor bone.[21] Where are the public health warnings regarding saliva?

It's not only a kiss that may infect. What if a spoon or a martini glass left on the counter carried the infective virus?

A 1985 report from the Pasteur Institute in Paris, France, revealed that concentrated *AIDS virus in saliva remains alive and infective on a dry surface at room temperature for as long as 7 days.*[22]

These studies were performed by allowing the virus to dry on a surface and then collecting a small specimen every few days and placing it in a test tube with human lymphocytes. Specimens collected after 7 days still were able to infect the lymphocytes with AIDS.

This study has been criticized because the virus in the saliva was in a higher concentration than is normally found in AIDS patients' saliva. Ryan White, before he died, spoke graphically on the Phil Donahue Show, "It would take an ocean of saliva to infect someone." He was wrong. There is no evidence that increased concentration of the virus causes an individual viral particle to live longer than usual. A higher concentration of the virus only improves the chances of finding a live particle in the specimen. It is reasonable to assume, at least until we have conclusive evidence to the contrary, that the virus really can survive under these circumstances, which would mean it is much more resistant to denaturing than previously believed.

Because sometimes a person is exposed to semen and blood in combination or semen and saliva in combination, or all three body fluids simultaneously, it is difficult to know which body fluid was responsible for transmission.

In a limited study, five homosexual men became HIV-positive as a result of oral sex. Two of the five participated in insertive fellatio only, which indicates that transmission was via saliva.[23]

The report states that this "was their only sexual practice, to the exclusion even of deep kissing." These findings suggest that saliva can be a vector for HIV in these circumstances.

It is impossible to ascertain whether the other three patients were infected by insertive or receptive fellatio, but it appears that oral sex is associated with a risk of transmission of HIV.

In a second study, Italian medical researchers analyzed the saliva of 45 healthy, uninfected heterosexual couples for blood cells in saliva. We know that blood cells transmit this virus. These researchers found that 55 percent of the couples had traces of blood in their saliva after eating. 80 percent showed traces of blood after brushing their teeth, and *91 percent after passionate kissing.*[24]

Most AIDS patients have weakened mucous membranes with inflamed gums and bleeding gum tissue. Logic tells you that in their saliva there would be blood cells in larger quantities than would be true of healthy people.

Transmission has also occurred from open wound to open wound where HIV-positive blood was spilled by accident.

For example, an American tourist in Africa became infected with the AIDS virus during a bus accident when blood from other injured passengers splashed into his wounds.

The 32 year old man had tested negative for the AIDS

virus when he donated blood just before he left for his trip. He had never used intravenous drugs and had no homosexual experiences. His heterosexual partners tested negative for the AIDS virus.[25]

A 25 year old Italian soccer player contracted the AIDS virus after an injury caused by a collision with another player during a soccer game.[26]

The Infectious Disease physician reported that the virus was apparently transmitted through severe cuts of the forehead sustained by *both players.*

Two months after the accident the player was found to be HIV-positive. One year before, he had tested negative and had no other risk factors.

The other man involved in the accident was a member of a soccer team composed of residents of a drug rehabilitation center and he had previously tested positive for HIV.

We have been told repeatedly that it takes an open wound for the virus to get into the bloodstream.

Apparently, that is not necessarily a requirement.

Research has shown that transmission does not require open wounds. HIV infection has occurred from infected blood coming in contact with intact mucous membranes and skin.

One example briefly cited in the previous chapter was a female phlebotomist who was splashed on the face and mouth with blood from a vacuum test tube. She had facial acne, but no open wounds. Although she cleaned the blood off immediately, she still turned HIV-positive.[27]

These findings seem to indicate that getting accidentally contaminated with blood on injured or even intact skin can lead to HIV infection. It is reasonable to assume from these cited incidents that AIDS can be contracted in any situation where blood of one individual can come into contact with skin or mucous membranes of another.

Such situations would include contact sports, accidents on a ski slope, or that car crash in your neighborhood where you rush in to pull a victim out.

Would they include the playground of your kindergartner?

And what about the sanitary napkins in a public rest room.

How about urine transmission? We know that the virus is present in urine. If it is there, it may transmit. The gay community keeps participating in what they call "golden showers" which means men urinate on other men for sexual arousal.

Is that high risk behavior? Nobody seems to know. Nobody seems to want to know.

The virus is present in tears, and ophthalmologists and opticians have been warned about the dangers of using the same trial contact lenses on more than one patient and to be scrupulous with storage fluid.[28]

Perspiration?

The Centers for Disease Control and the former Surgeon General have been adamant in their assertion that AIDS cannot be transmitted by sweat. You would think that if they were making such a statement, they would have some facts to back up their assertion.

I asked Dr. Adelissa Panlillio of the CDC less than a year ago if the virus was present in perspiration.

"This could be a problem on the equipment in gyms," I pointed out to her.

She told me energetically, "No. No. The virus is not present in sweat."

I asked her for her references.

She said to me with visible impatience, "Well, if it were in sweat, everybody would have the disease, wouldn't they?"

There are many diseases that are known to be transmitted in specific ways, yet not all those exposed to the disease will contract the disease. Tuberculosis can be transmitted by coughing, but not everyone has TB.

I said to Adelissa, "I'd like to see the research. Why don't you just give me the articles proving that HIV can't be found in perspiration?"

She responded, "Well, we have no recorded cases of it being transmitted by sweat."

I exclaimed, "But, you have published that you are not even looking. Your studies look only at transmission through blood. How can you say that there are no recorded cases when you are not even looking? The first thing we need to know is whether or not the virus is present in sweat."

She finally admitted, "Well, we don't know. Nobody has looked at it."

I said: "Why, then, do you tell the American public that the AIDS virus it is not present in sweat?"

AIDSpeak is glib in skirting the issue.

The CDC authorities do not come out and tell you categorically: "The virus is not present in perspiration." They will tell you: "There are *no recorded cases* of it being transmitted that way."

If you assume that means that the virus is not there, they'll let you.

When I talked to Dr. James Curran, who is Dr. Panlillio's

superior, and related this verbal exchange to him later, I asked him, "Why is she allowed to say that? And why does the Centers for Disease Control hold the stance that AIDS can't be transmitted through sweat when you really don't know?"

He said, "You know how it is. Adelissa is young, and when you are young, it is very difficult to say 'I don't know.'"

I still want to know if the virus is present in perspiration. Don't you?

I understand that some work has been done in France, but I have not been able to track down the source.

I want to make it very clear that I am not saying that AIDS can be transmitted by a handshake. I am just objecting to the AIDSpeak dictum that it can't.

I'd like to know, first, is it present in sweat?

Secondly, if so, what is the concentration of the virus present.

And finally, just how many viral particles are needed to infect?

Let's put one myth to rest: HIV is *not* a "fragile" virus.

It is a remarkably hardy virus. Not all disinfectants will kill it. Maybe not even most.

Do the American people generally, and health care workers specifically, know that:

*   The virus is not inactivated by 70 percent ethyl alcohol poured on it for twenty minutes?

At the Montreal AIDS Convention in June of 1989, it was shown that the virus when dried in body fluids would not be inactivated if it was treated with ethyl alcohol for twenty minutes.[29] Dried virus is what health care workers deal with after an operation when blood and other body fluids are deposited on instruments. It's dried blood on the linens. It's dried blood on the floor.

* Certain chemicals used for sterilizing instruments that cannot be autoclaved will not deactivate the virus?

Scopes used to look inside the abdomen or joints, for example, cannot be put up to high heat because of their delicate instrumentation. These instruments are put in what we call "cold sterilization"—chemical sterilization. One of those common sterilization fluids is called glutaraldehyde. It has been found by the same researchers, that 1 percent glutaraldehyde will not inactivate the dried AIDS virus over twenty minutes, but 2 percent glutaraldehyde will.

We have been told that virtually all antiseptics and household detergents will inactivate the virus. Those studies were done with the virus in liquid suspension, not dried in body fluids. We now know that the virus, when dried in body fluids, is much more resistant to inactivation.

Does Clorox kill the virus? I don't know. I have seen the study that was referred to me by the CDC purporting to show that Clorox kills the virus. The study is impossible to decipher. Even if good studies exist, we would still have to ask: Were those studies done with the virus wet or dried? Were the findings replicated elsewhere? Did the compound kill all of the virus of just 50 percent of it, as is the end-point in many studies.

And finally, here are a couple of thought-provoking experiments that show that "intact" skin is not a barrier.

In 1976, it was discovered by scientists specializing in dermatology that a specific cell called the Langerhans cell in the skin was the target cell for external contact allergens—that is, these cells were responsible for what we call an allergic reaction in that they attached to the irritant particle and transported it through the skin and gave it to the cell that started the allergic reaction.[30]

Langerhans cells are found tightly packed in mucous membranes and more loosely distributed in all human skin.

A few years ago these Langerhans cells were examined to see if they have attachments for the HIV virus, called CD4 receptors.

Researchers isolated a number of Langerhans cells, put them in a test tube and added HIV virus to see if it would attach to the cells. And, sure enough, it did. The Langerhans cells have receptors specific for HIV.[31] This means that cells in your skin and mucous membranes are capable of "recognizing" the virus and attaching to it.

The next question the researchers asked was, "Can HIV be transmitted through intact skin or intact mucous membranes?"

Dr. Llasa Braathen, from Bern, Switzerland, investigated the answer to this question. Here, briefly, is his ingenious experiment:

He took what was felt to be intact skin into the laboratory and put semen infected with HIV on top of the intact skin. Before he did that, he made the HIV "visible" by tagging it with a fluorescent compound so it could be photographed with a special camera.[32]

He watched as the Langerhans cells, which have long finger-like fine extensions, transported the HIV down into the lower layers of the skin. *The fluorescent HIV was now no longer on top of the skin, but within the skin, which shows that skin is not a sufficient barrier.*

The problem with the evidence above is that the research has not been publicized. Much of the troubling "evidence" that HIV may be transmitted in ways other than the "accepted and acknowledged ways" is either not acknowledged or deliberately ridiculed.

Somebody has seen smoke. It could have come from anywhere.

AIDSpeak decries the "unscientific" inference of fire.

Yet facts, said Aldous Huxley, don't cease to exist because they are ignored.

Just recently, at the 1991 AIDS International Conference in Florence Italy, Dr. William Hazeltine presented "new" evidence that HIV can be transmitted through *intact* mucous membranes via Langerhans cells. When Dr. Llasa Braathen said it years ago, nobody listened.

There has been enormous philosophical and political resistance to the very idea of casual contact transmission.

We all have heard heart-warming stories of kind-hearted people who have taken castaway AIDS babies into their homes, hugged them, kissed them, burped them, changed their diapers, cuddled them against bare skin—all this to the triumphant conclusion that "not one of them has ever fallen ill."

Will this be true ten years from now?

That these kind souls who cuddle their infected babies without adequate protection are not yet ill today is not convincing "proof" that it will not happen tomorrow.

Barbara Bush and Princess Diana hug AIDS-infected

babies to prove it's not dangerous. They get their information from the "experts" mentioned in this book who have been wrong many times.

At the beginning of the AIDS epidemic several studies were done to evaluate the possiblity of household transmission, studies that all concluded that transmission by household contact did not happen. According to the "experts," people who lived with HIV-infected victims did not turn HIV-positive.[33,34]

Most of this research involved cross-sectional studies—that is, comparisons "on the spot" of HIV households to non-HIV households. Only a few household members were ever studied over time.

To my knowledge, that time span has never been longer than 12 months. Apparently, not one of these studies is being continued.

After attending the 1989 AIDS Conference in Montreal, I checked with Dr. Curran of the Centers for Disease Control.

I said, "I can't find any abstracts from presentations on continuing household contact studies. Did I miss them? I can check my abstract booklet again."

He told me, "No, there are no more household contact studies continuing."

Let me repeat this warning once more for the record:

The "negative window" is three-and-a-half years. Sometimes a body needs that long to show that infection has occurred.

It can take ten years or more for an infected victim to develop full-blown AIDS.

Thus, only testing over time would give a more accurate picture.

Watch AIDSpeak in action the next time you pick up a paper. The buzz phrase is, "No Identified Risk Factor." Consistently, 3-5 percent of all AIDS cases reported, including children, have "No Identified Risk Factor.

In other words, these people didn't get AIDS in any of the usual ways the government admits AIDS can be transmitted, such as through homosexual sex, sharing dirty needles, blood transfusions or from infected mother to baby at birth. That means that after thorough investigation, the public health authorities don't know how the patient got AIDS. It strongly suggests to me as it may suggest to you, that there are other ways AIDS can be transmitted.

In 1989, diagnosed AIDS cases increased by 14 percent compared with 1988. Of the total number of AIDS cases, 5.2 percent had no identified risk factors.[35]

That 5.2 percent represents 1,848 persons with "No Identified Risk Factors" in 1989, an increase from 1,012 in 1988.

That is a 55 percent increase in only one year of people who contracted the disease and no one knows how.

7

I Quit!

Day: ". . . if you came to work every day and flipped the light switch on in your office, and only one out of 200 times you were electrocuted, would you consider that low-risk?"

Kroft: "The people at this hospital—for the most part, the administrators—say that you are suffering essentially from what they call AIDS anxiety."

Day: "Oh! Well! I guess I am suffering from AIDS anxiety! I think that if you were faced with a fatal disease every single day when you went to work . . . you would have a certain amount of anxiety. It is appropriate. It's called survival."

Voice-over: "There are six and a half million health care workers in the United States and, according to the Centers for Disease Control here in Atlanta, there are only 18 documented cases of on-the-job infection. Those numbers have been used to try and persuade health care workers that their chances of getting the virus on the job are low."

Day: "How did they come up with those figures? Did they test all 6.5 million health care workers? They've tested a very small percentage. . ."

Kroft: "You think the CDC is underplaying the threat."

Day: "Absolutely. Absolutely."

Voice-over: "In fact, no one really believes the figure of 18 health care workers infected—including Dr. Jim Curran of the CDC.

Curran: "It's certainly much more than 18. And probably much less than several hundred."

Voice-over: "Dr. Curran is in charge of the AIDS program at the Centers for Disease Control. He acknowledges that relatively few health care workers have been tested, but insists the documented infection rate is small. He does concede some workers face more risks than others."

Curran: "I think that surgeons and people who have a substantial amount of needlesticks and cuts during surgery have a considerable potential of infection from blood-borne infections, including HIV as well as hepatitis B."

Kroft: "We asked the question to Lorraine Day, and she said, 'Absolutely. It's high-risk behavior. My chances of contracting the AIDS virus from one needlestick are greater than they are from having anal sex, or gay sex.'"

Curran (hesitating): "They're probably about the same. The needlestick from an AIDS patient versus one sexual contact *with anal intercourse."*

Kroft: "So you're saying the risks are pretty high."

Curran: "Significant. I think the risks are something that have to be dealt with. . ."

Kroft: "Most health care workers we spoke with were under the impression that the CDC does not consider their risks significant. And as recently as April of 1988, the CDC published a report which warned health care workers to be careful with blood, but also reported that the occupational risk of acquiring HIV in a health care setting is low."

Curran: "I don't think that characterizing the risk as low is accurate. I believe that the risk for someone who gets a needlestick is a substantial one, and one should be concerned."

Kroft: "Are you guilty of underplaying the risks to medical workers?"

Curran: "I don't like to dwell on the past so much as to deal with what has to happen in the future. I don't feel any guilt. . ."

Excerpt from a *60 Minutes* segment with Steve Kroft,
September 24, 1989
© CBS Inc. 1989 All Rights Reserved.

It's not just needlesticks.

It's attitudes. It's negligence. It's intimidation. It's taking us for granted when we are putting our lives right on the line. It's lack of understanding about what happens in a health care setting, particularly in the operating room when we are dealing with patients who have AIDS.

AIDS has profoundly changed the working atmosphere for health care personnel. From the gay community, it's confrontation now. It's power politics. It's short term gains at the expense of long term tragedy.

This atmosphere makes it difficult to want to serve in a profession most of us chose because we felt we had a mission, and it will get much worse before it will get better.

It has been argued vigorously in AIDSpeak parlance that health care workers *know* their work is hazardous. It is believed that they are, in a way, born to take great risks.

After all, have they not always been at risk for hepatitis?

For example, some 300 health care workers per year are known to die from hepatitis B contracted in the workplace. Prior to the AIDS epidemic, it was never argued that all health care workers should be noble, close both eyes, accept their risks of getting hepatitis and get on with their business of being selfless citizens.

For years and years, potential infection from hepatitis B was nobody's private agenda. The infectious disease specialists were not campaigning to warn health care workers of their risk. Hepatitis took center stage only after infection via HIV became a political issue. Now the infectious disease specialists cite our prior risks of hepatitis as if those prior risks now justify our current and our future risks from HIV. It cannot be logically argued that a person who might get killed by a car out of control should stand still in the path of a truck.

The risk of infection from hepatitis B compared to the risk of infection from HIV are not comparable risks.

Not only will hepatitis infection lead to death in only one

percent of all infections that occur, but also there now exists a safe and effective vaccine to prevent hepatitis. Furthermore, treatment for hepatitis is readily available. For years most health care workers have accepted the risk of infection from hepatitis as part of their job. They may not have liked the odds against them, but they have accepted them. They have never asked for a risk-free environment.

But HIV is always fatal.

There is no vaccine.

There is only token treatment for AIDS that can slow down the disease and delay ultimate death by only a few months.

All right. So there is danger, but there also is danger in crossing the street. We can't have a life without danger. Therefore, "Just be careful," we are told, and furthermore "If you do get a needlestick, it's your own fault for being clumsy."

Health care workers have been told innumerable times that being "careful" in handling contaminated people or items will eliminate the danger of contracting AIDS. Avoiding direct contact with body fluids and accidental injuries, AIDSpeak announces everywhere, will virtually eliminate the risk.

Thinking the problem will be solved by telling people to be careful is simplistic. If that approach had any merit, we could eliminate all traffic accidents by telling people to be careful on the roads. We could eliminate all hip fractures in the elderly by telling them not to fall down. And if these accidents happen, should we just blame it on the poor elderly people who fell down?

The risk to health care workers is substantial. In documenting that risk, let's start at the top, where risk is believed to be highest.

It has been documented, but not widely publicized, that specific occupations within the health care industry carry an enormous risk. Viral laboratory workers, for example, are particularly vulnerable, according to the Office of Safety and Health Administration (OSHA). The chances of contracting AIDS in a viral lab are nearly 20 percent over a 45-year working lifetime, reports OSHA.

> "For research and production laboratory workers with occupational exposure to high concentrations of the (AIDS) virus," states an OSHA entry in the Federal Register, "the risk of seroconversion . . . over a 45 year working lifetime would be 195 per 1000 exposed workers"[1]

What's buried in the obtuse language above is this: a ghastly and premature death for one in every five viral lab workers!

That's madness.

What industry would hold still to a one-in-five risk of death from a specific occupational disease? If one waitress in five would die of cancer due to secondary smoke inhalation, we wouldn't allow smoking in restaurants. If there were a one-in-five chance your child might die in a bus accident, you wouldn't send your child to school in a bus. Would we have many pilots flying our planes if one in five would crash? Would passengers use airplanes?

That is the kind of risk some workers are asked to take.

It's very simple, really. It's unacceptable.

"But," say the skeptics. "Working in a viral lab is laboring in an exceptionally hazardous environment. Some firemen die in a fire. Some astronauts die in explosions."

Yes, accidents may happen especially in some occupations that are riskier than others. Being an astronaut is very risky business. Being a fireman is extremely dangerous.

But do we give a fireman a T-shirt and shorts and say, "Now go and save somebody?"

Do we send an astronaut into the sky to risk his life without protective gear? Do we rocket him up into the air without first having spent millions in perfecting heat-resistant tiles for the space capsule to make sure he returns safely to earth?

The watch words in our space programs are maximum resources, efficiency of mission, investigation of risk and prevention of the perils of an accident. Our astronauts are valuable. The money allocated to them is put up front, not set aside for accidents. Prevention is the goal, not care of casualties. The people at the hub are scientists. They aren't bureaucrats.

Our astonauts are valuable and so are our firemen. American taxpayers are willing to give them whatever equipment and training they need to do their jobs appropriately and safely.

American health care workers, however, are taken for granted. Why is that so? Because there is more glamour in going to the stars or putting out a fire than there might be in emptying a bedpan at less than $5 an hour?

Both astronauts and nurses' aides, within their specialties, are trying hard to make this a better world. And we need both. As individuals, we may well need a nurses' aide before we need an astronaut. What will we do if nurses' aides take flight?

The risk to them is real, and the public health authorities must admit it. This message must sink in. American leaders will respond to the mandate of safety for high risk professions if they believe the risk is real. They will not respond to that mandate if the risk is perceived to be low.

We need protective gear. We need it now. We cannot do without it. The virus will as surely act on an unprotected health care worker as gravity acts on a falling spaceship. Unless there is a safety net, there's going to be a crash.

It was a Saturday.

I was called in to care for a known AIDS patient who had a massive infection of his foot—simply a huge wound. I could take my gloved hand and tunnel from his heel all the way down to his toes under the skin of his foot. He had a temperature of almost 106°. He was a very sick man when I saw him, and time was of the essence. He needed to have that area cleaned up, and we were afraid we were going to have to amputate his foot unless we acted fast and furiously.

My young chief resident, Dr. Michelle James, and I were going to go in to the operating room and treat this case to save this man's foot if not his life.

We knew that the patient had AIDS.

In order to irrigate the infected area, we had to use an intermittent spray, which is like a water pick, a device that splashes pus and blood all over. At that time we were unaware of the need for spacesuits.

There are little plastic umbrellas, however, that go over the spraying nozzle to cut down on the splatter. They are cheap and disposable costing perhaps $5 each. That weekend, the hospital was all out of those little shields and they had been on back order for some time.

I said, "We are not going to do this without those umbrellas. It is too dangerous because it will spray back at us."

The answer was, "Well, Dr. Day, we don't have any."

I responded, "Then you will go right now to another hospital, please, and you will borrow a supply for us. I am not going in there, and I am not allowing my chief resident to go in there without one. And may I please point out that this patient needs to have treatment. Now."

So off went someone, pouting all the way.

Of course there was a big delay. We waited. We waited some more. She came back, finally, and said, "Here, we have five."

I said, "I am on call this weekend. I may have 20 patients coming in who need to have this kind of irrigation procedure."

At that point the head nurse responded in a voice just half an inch short of sedition, "Well, then I guess you will just have to use them on your worst patients, Dr. Day."

But see? That brings me back to Chapter I. How do I know who is my "worst" patient? I'm not allowed to know.

Here is another example that happened at the University of California, San Francisco, which is a teaching hospital.

I had recently turned in my letter of resignation as Chief of Orthopedic Surgery at San Francisco and had just quit operating there. I had transferred my operating procedures to U.C. hospital because my risk of being infected with AIDS in a trauma hospital in San Francisco was too high. My supervisors had asked me to stay on as Chief of Orthopedic Surgery until they found my replacement. I continued my administrative duties at San Francisco General hospital and decided that I would operate in a lower risk setting such as the University hospital to see if I wanted to continue working as an orthopedic surgeon at all.

One of my first patients in the new setting was a young, gay, HIV-infected man. When I walked into the examining room, we had the following exchange:

"I recognize you. You are Dr. Day."

"Yes, I am."

"You used to be at San Francisco General Hospital."

"That's correct."

"I heard you speak on AIDS at the Hyatt."

"Oh?"

I looked at the man, and I assessed that he was probably gay. As it turned out, he was also a diabetic and he told me he was HIV-positive.

We started talking rather pleasantly about his orthopedic problem. He had swelling of the wrist causing pressure on the nerve to his hand, a condition called carpal tunnel syndrome, that can be treated short-term by injections with cortisone, which can decrease the inflammation and the swelling and, thereby, decrease the pressure on the nerve.

But too many cortisone injections in one area can cause tissue breakdown and eventually lead to infection, particularly in a diabetic. And, of course, a physician is always worried about an infection in an HIV-positive patient.

Therefore I said to this patient, "I think it is unwise to continue injections into your wrist because you have had eight already from other doctors. As you have just confirmed, the benefits of injection last only a few months, and then the pain returns. It's better that you have an operation. I can release the carpal ligament. It can be done as a come-and-go procedure, and your problem will be solved permanently."

I could tell he was hesitant about having the operation. Since I knew he was aware that my name was attached to a great deal of controversy regarding AIDS, I said to him, "Would you prefer to have another doctor operate on you?"

"You mean you *would* operate on me?"

"Only if you want me to."

"Then I will have the operation," said the patient, "if you will do it."

"I will do it."

"If you think I need an operation and you are willing to do it, then I know I need an operation."

"Fine."

I told him he had to have one other study done. He should come back in a week and we would schedule the operation. I recorded this information in his chart, then I related this conversation to the nurse, who is head of the clinic, because I thought it was unusual that a gay, HIV-positive patient clearly aware of my incorrect image as a "homophobic" doctor wanted me to do the operation. I also thought that was the end of it.

When I went back to the clinic a few days later, I was informed that this man had called repeatedly, complaining bitterly, telling the head nurse and others in the clinic, "Dr. Day refused to inject my wrist because I am HIV-positive." Fortunately the head nurse knew the whole story and refused to allow the patient to continue with such incorrect statements.

Here I was trying to decrease my dangers by changing hospitals, yet I was willing to put myself at higher risk by performing an operation that was clearly much more dangerous to me than simply injecting the wrist, but an operation that was better for the patient. Even so, my treatment and my strategy were challenged as discrimination against an AIDS patient.

Incidents like these two make for a great deal of resentment in a health care setting where professionals are doing their best to treat AIDS patients without having physical safety and moral support. Nothing in the AIDSpeak business is so unfair and so untrue as is the widely held belief that health care workers are at "low risk" and unwilling to put themselves on the line.

Low risk? Compared to whom? Compared with what?

Unprotected vaginal sex with a HIV-positive partner carries a risk of one in 500 for contracting HIV per single occurrence.[2]

Unprotected anal intercourse with a known HIV-positive partner has a documented risk of transmitting the infection of one in 250.[3]

Yet according to the Centers for Disease Control. a single needlestick with HIV-positive blood carries a risk of getting AIDS of one in 200-250.

And that risk is not just a cumulative risk, the way radiation exposure would be: the fatal stick can be the very first one!

At my hospital, orthopedic surgeons—and now others—wear protective gear when doing surgery on AIDS patients as though they were going into battle which is, in fact, what they are doing. Every time we go into the operating room, we do the following:

We wear double shoe covers over knee-high, water-resistant boots. We don disposable reinforced gowns. We wear additional sleeve covers. We have full-face protection such as face shields. We wear double or triple latex gloves or fabric gloves between two latex gloves to increase protection against cuts. We have respirator industrial masks available for use as needed. While operating on high risk patients we wear our *notorious* "space suits" to filter out bloody aersosls.

At San Francisco General Hospital a system has been developed to aid a health care worker who has received a needlestick. We follow emergency protocol. Here's what we suggest a health care worker do as soon as contamination has occurred:

* Immediately remove gloves and "bleed" the wound.

* Thoroughly wash the wound with soap and water. We do not recommend pouring Clorox on the wound because Clorox is caustic and may make the skin more vulnerable to later exposure to hazardous blood or other body fluids.

* A doctor or nurse from the Infectious Disease Division who carries a "needlestick beeper" can be contacted any time of day or night to authorize the pharmacy to provide AZT to the injured health care worker.

Although, there are no animal or human studies indicating that AZT will decrease the chances of becoming HIV-positive, there is a suggestion that it may delay the onset of symptoms for a time.

Because AZT has significant side effects, including nausea, vomiting and anemia individuals taking the drug must be followed by a physician and must weigh the pros and cons before deciding on this course of treatment.

Other emergency crews have followed suit similarly. Because our protocol has proven helpful and expedient, it has been imitated by other health care systems.

For example, firefighters, police officers and health care workers exposed to the AIDS virus on the job now can get AZT free in a new program initiated by Orange County, California. We have had inquiries from many other associations, corporations and organizations.

These measures are speculative, however, because there is still no evidence this protocol actually changes the outcome. Either we turn HIV-positive or we don't. It's still Russian roulette.

Needlesticks are only one of many dangers from HIV-infected patients that health care workers face.

As previously stated, Officials from the Centers for Disease Control have admitted, that the virus can be found in many body fluids. The occupational risks of coming in contact with urine, feces, sputum, tears, vomitus, semen and other body fluids are presently unknown.

Partly because of weak research design and partly for lack of personnel, lack of money and lack of intellectual curiosity, there aren't even estimates as to how high that risk might be. There aren't even guesses.

Many health care workers, especially in an emergency, will work with their bare hands even in cases in which the virus is present and active. Chances are that it will infect. In a high risk battlefield such as a hospital, chances are there will be casualties.

For example, health care workers are largely unaware that the amount of virus contained in saliva has been sufficient to have caused transmission in unorthodox ways. Most health care workers worry only about blood.

But even setting the question of non-blood transmission aside for now and focusing only on blood, we hear over and over that the risk to health care workers is low.

The AIDSpeak myth of "low risk" obscures a real and present danger to health care workers and allied professions. Unfortunately, it is delivered with remarkable conviction even by some of the health care workers themselves, the ones who serve where the fires are hottest. I often hear the platitude that "millions and millions of health care workers are being exposed to AIDS every day, and only a tiny fraction have turned positive. . . ."

But how do we know that? How many have been tested? We cannot make such statements because we aren't counting and extrapolating properly. "Given a thimbleful of facts," says Gordon Allport, "we rush to make generalizations as large as a tub."

In interviews and press releases officials of the Centers for Disease Control have stated repeatedly that, so far, there are "less than 40 health care workers with no other risk factors" who have turned HIV-positive from occupational exposure.

Even granted that this number is correct—and, as we now surmise, it probably is not, since there are serious discrepancies in numbers even within the various factions of the same federal bureaucracies—how many health care workers who have been exposed have had repeated tests for HIV?

Only a very few.

We must remember also that not all of the nation's health care workers have yet come in contact with AIDS. In fact, more health care workers probably have not yet had direct exposure to AIDS patients than those who have. AIDS incidence is still pretty concentrated in several large cities such as New York, Los Angeles and San Francisco.

But even those who have been exposed are not being monitored closely. Chances are they are excluded from the "occupational transmission" category if they also have a "high-risk lifestyle." Chances are they are excluded if they were not tested before exposure. Chances are that even if they have been tested, they aren't being followed up long enough, a critical consideration, given the "negative window" factor.

"Guidelines for Prevention of HIV and Hepatitis to Health Care and Public Safety Workers," published by the CDC in June of 1989, reveals that only 2,396 health care workers are known to have been tested. Of these, six were HIV-positive. The CDC also lists another 22 health care workers who have turned positive after a specific event of exposure to HIV-positive blood.[4]

Please note the selectivity of this sample.

These are health care employees who actually reported the injury and were screened out in terms of "other-risk" factors. They turned antibody positive within the designated period of time. They were "fortunate" enough to have had a documented negative test prior to HIV exposure.

This sample does not include those health care workers with injuries that do not get reported. It does not count the ones who may report but are dismissed as having "other" high risk factors that might have caused HIV infection. It does not acknowledge the ones who have become HIV positive but have a longer incubation time and may not show up positive on the antibody test for many months or several years.

Below are the dubious findings of another governmental agency.

The Department of Labor's Occupational Safety and Health Administration published a *Federal Register* entry on May 30, 1989, beginning on page 23,055 that discusses in detail 25 cases of occupational exposure. Five pages into the report, we learn that there was "further evidence of occupational transmission" in additional health care workers. As of September 19, 1989, there were in fact, 169 workers in this group.

We are told, that data collected is incomplete for 28 of these health care workers because of death or refusal to be interviewed. Investigations are in progress for 97 others, and case investigations have been completed for the remaining 44 persons.

Among the latter there are eight physicians, including four surgeons, one dentist, six nurses, nine nursing assistants, eight housekeeping or maintenance workers, four clinical laboratory technicians, two therapists, one mortician, one paramedic, and four others "who did not have contact with patients." That is a smorgasboard across a wide spectrum of health-related professions who all had some form of occupational exposure and have become contaminated.

Did all of them contaminate themselves by means of needlesticks or by only coming in contact with blood, for that matter?

When officials of the Centers for Disease Control reported that there were "less than 20 known cases," they did not count the casualties just listed: 25 plus an additional 44 health care workers whose pending investigation has now been completed, plus several dozen "likely" casualties *for a total of approximately 100 who have no other risk factors for AIDS and who are HIV-positive.*

The CDC readily admits that the number of health care workers infected with AIDS, that they are aware of, is grossly underestimated.

And what is so ironic is that the struggle for protection for those very workers is met with an assault on our professional integrity.

Not long after I started speaking out on behalf of greater health care safety, I found myself being investigated behind my back by San Francisco General Hospital's Quality Assurance Committee on whether or not I had "denied care" to AIDS patients.

To the best of my knowledge, this type of investigation had never been conducted covertly in any instance for any reason to any other surgeon or doctor *ever* in the entire history of the hospital.

Eventually, I was called in, without even knowing the names of the patients I was supposed to have wronged. The committee that was assembled included not one professional who had anything to do with orthopedic surgery.

A paper with the patients' names had been passed out to everyone. I was told that two patients on my service had been denied care because they were HIV-positive.

I asked the committee chairman to please tell me about them.

As it turned out, they were not even personal patients of mine; they were patients of people on my staff. However, since the patients on my service are all under my supervisory care and since I keep a close watch on all patients of the staff I supervise, I did remember them.

The first was a young woman drug addict, infected with the AIDS virus, who had a massive infection in her hip. She was demanding to have a total hip replacement.

Every orthopedic surgeon knows that you do not put a plastic-and-metal hip prosthesis into the infected hip joint of a drug addict who is continuing to shoot drugs irrespective of whether or not they are infected with HIV. Street drugs are often contaminated with bacteria that can get into the blood-stream and can cause infection any place in the body. The bacteria are particularly attracted to the plastic and metal of the artificial hip. Pus in the hip of an HIV-positive patient with immune suppression problems, furthermore, would have guaranteed the hip replacement surgery ultimately to fail. Even if she had been HIV-negative, she still would not have qualified for total hip replacement because of the severe infection in her hip.

After I explained all that to the committee, they reluctantly decided that there had not been denial of care.

The next case was an alcoholic HIV-infected patient who had a recurrent posterior dislocation of his shoulder. Ninety-five percent of all shoulder dislocations are anterior in direction of dislocation. If you see someone with a posterior dislocation, the most common cause is seizures. This patient had seizures from his alcoholism; moreover, he was refusing to take his anti-seizure medication.

All orthopedic surgeons know that a person who has uncontrolled seizures is not a candidate for shoulder repair surgery. If surgery is performed, when the patient wakes up from his anesthetic, he can have a grand mal seizure which causes his entire operative repair to rip open.

I explained all that to the committee, too. They came to the conclusion that there was no denial of care with that case either.

Both cases had nothing to do with the patients' HIV status. Each decision had been a medical one made in the patient's best interest.

I asked the chairman of the committee to destroy the

inaccurate memo that had charged me with denial of care so that it wouldn't get distributed to others in the hospital.

He told me that it would be done. But it was not done. This memo saying that I stood accused of having denied care to AIDS-afflicted patients was distributed—perhaps accidentally, perhaps on purpose—to every surgeon in the Department of Surgery.

The newspapers got hold of it and then the story went from coast to coast. Other papers picked it up. AIDSpeak was having a field day.

Recently, when I was in England, I heard this accusation there.

It is small wonder that more doctors don't speak out on this issue.

After I became aware of the enormous danger to me and my staff via exposure to blood and other body fluids, I had packed a suitcase full of orthopedic instruments and gone over to the University hospital to pay a visit to the Chancellor, Dr. Julius Krevans. Because Dr. Krevans is an internal medicine doctor, not a surgeon, I wanted to show him how sharp and, hence, dangerous my surgical instruments were.

I actually stuck his hand with a few K-wires as I told him, "These are sharp! These are what we work with. I want you to know that we think we are at great risk, not just from needlesticks but from all kinds of surgical instruments. My staff, my residents, my nurses and I are in danger. We need someone important who is in a decision-making capacity to be responsible for our safety from AIDS. I don't ever want to be accused of not going through channels."

As I remember it, he told me he was interested in the problem; he would look into it.

Some time after my visit, the aforementioned aerosol article appeared in the *Journal of the American Medical Association*[5] showing that laser beams, when applied to a genital wart, were aerosolizing the human papilloma virus in the laser smoke plume, keeping it airborne indefinitely. Laser users were warned that a regular surgical mask would not protect them.

The *Clinical Laser Monthly* came out shortly thereafter with much the same information, stating that even though transmission by aerosols had not yet been proved, prudence was the wisest course. Surgeons and other operating room personnel should wear a respirator, not just a surgical mask.

When I read that, my radar started quivering. Could it be possible to breathe in HIV from aerosols?

I thought, "What are we doing in the operating room when we are drilling and reaming on bloody HIV-positive bone with our power instruments? We are using high-speed drills and high-speed saws. Blood is flying everywhere! Even though people seem to think that HIV is very fragile, is it possible that it could be infective in the aerosols we are creating surgically?"

I wrote a letter to the Chancellor, in which I included copies of the documented evidence of potential risk.

I said in this letter, in part, "I think we need to investigate whether or not we are aerosolizing HIV. I will continue to do all emergency operations on all patients. I will even do all semi-emergent operations. But I want to postpone regularly scheduled elective operations on known HIV-positive or high-risk patients until we can scientifically check out if bloody aerosols are produced in the operating room."

This was not in any way a revolutionary request.

We postpone elective surgery all the time because we are the area's only trauma hospital. Routine electively scheduled operations are bumped off of the schedule because of the many emergencies we have.

No patient would be harmed by such a decision.

I took great care in drafting this letter because I did not want to spend another year tiptoeing across more political mine fields, given the preceding controversy over wanting to do voluntary testing for HIV and the resulting fury from both colleagues, lay people and the press.

I stated clearly in my letter that I was not refusing to operate on any HIV-positive or HIV-suspect patients. I just wanted to postpone non-urgent surgery until we had tested the bloody air in the operating room to see if we needed additional protection. I said I felt it was my moral duty to investigate, not only for myself, but for the other young doctors I was training and the nurses in the operating room, some of whom were pregnant.

I was called in by the University of California Associate Dean at San Francisco General Hospital, Dr. Elliot Rapaport who told me bluntly that it was unacceptable to postpone routine elective operations on HIV-positive or HIV-suspect patients. If I did not rescind my letter, said Dr. Rappaport, he herewith gave me notice that the administrator of the hospital would take out papers to have me replaced as Chief of the Orthopedic Surgery Service.

I looked at him and said, "Elliot, don't you care about the lives of health care workers? Don't you care?"

He told me that he cared, but what I was proposing was still unacceptable.

I said to him, "Even if you don't care about the lives of health care workers, don't you care about money? If a health care worker turns positive and sues the University, Elliot, it may cost you millions."

That potent argument did not persuade him either. He said again that my idea of postponement was not one he as a hospital dean could allow.

In response, true to my style and my conviction, I replied, "I am sorry, Elliot. That is the way it is. Aerosols have to be investigated, and I will not rescind my letter."

Later on, Dr. Rapaport denied before others that he had threatened my job. When I took this matter to the Academic Senate, he claimed that he was only trying to *let me know* "as a friend" what might happen to me if I kept up my stubborn demand.

That's not, however, how Elliot came across to me in this first confrontation. I stood up, locked eyes with him, and told him, "When you have those papers ready to have me removed as Chief of the Orthopedic Surgery Service for wanting greater safety in my work environment, give me ten copies for my attorneys, please."

What happened next could have been easily predicted.

I am told that the U.C. Dean, Dr. Rudi Schmid went to my own department chairman, Dr. William Murray, and told him, "If you can't get her to rescind her letter, we are going to remove all funding from your entire department!"

That's mayhem to any department chairman. It spells the doom for his department.

Bill Murray did not take that lying down. He thought up a creative solution. Up until that time he had not been a strong supporter of mine, but as fate would have it, a couple of his patients who were infected with HIV needed total hip replacements. He himself was going to be at risk for HIV because he was now going to be creating his own aerosols in the operating room.

Bill, therefore, offered me $50,000 of set-aside departmental funds to begin research on aerosols.

I promised to go by state-of-siege rules and hold my fire as long as we could at least begin to investigate whether bloody aerosols are dangerous.

By this time, I was growing weary of the intimidation and felt it should stop.

I thought the crucial issue for me was academic freedom. Officials from both the University and San Francisco General Hospital had tried to intimidate me again and again, first with the *Nightline* interview where I was not allowed to speak inside the hospital building, then the malpractice insurance threat, the Quality Assurance investigation and now this new aerosol matter with the threat to my job.

I fortified myself with solid documentation and research and went up to talk to Dr. Pete Ralston who was President of the Academic Senate to find out the proper University committee to handle my grievance.

After a great deal of talking, he decided it would be the Privilege and Tenure Committee. So, armed with thirteen sets of papers, I went over to talk to the Chairman of the Privilege and Tenure Committee, Dr. Ken Dill.

I asked Dr. Dill, "Is this committee going to be strong enough to handle this explosive matter? I am entitled to freedom of speech and academic freedom, and I intend to show that I am right in what I have been saying. But even if I were wrong, I have the right to speak.

"I have been saying that there is risk to health care workers, and I have found myself being prevented from speaking out on that risk. If you end up deciding in my favor, you are going to have to censure your own Dean, Dr. Rudi Schmid. The Dean is your boss! Are you and your committee going to be strong enough to censure your own boss?"

Dr. Dill answered me, "If this committee is not strong enough to do that, Dr. Day, then the committee members have no right to be on this committee. So, yes, in answer to your question, we can do that. If we have to do it, we'll censure our own boss."

I said, "That's great. That's wonderful. I feel better already."

I presented my concerns about my academic freedom to the Privilege and Tenure Committee. I gave them all the information I thought relevant. Then I waited. And waited. And waited.

Finally, I called Dr. Dill who told me that Dr. Schmid, the Dean, was "too busy" to appear, but that Dr. Rapaport, the Associate Dean, had been called in to talk to the Privilege and Tenure Committee.

It seems that Dr. Rapaport told the committee members, in so many words, that I must have misunderstood. How could I have gotten that idea? Nobody had abridged my academic freedom. No one was impeding my freedom of speech. No one was trying to threaten me. I was just being warned what would happen to me. The suggestion was that I had misunderstood the entire conversation.

Let me say here that when my superior warns me about what will happen to my job if I persist, that to me is a threat.

I also learned a very important political rule, namely, if you are trying to intimidate somebody, don't ever write it down.

Dr. Rapaport had not written anything down, and apparently made that point to the committee. There was no paper trail.

The university lawyer, Joe Cowan, had not written anything down pertaining to his threat that I would not be covered by malpractice insurance.

Finally, after several months, Dr. Dill informed me that his committee was not the proper forum for this grievance, even though the President of the Academic Senate, after much investigation had directed me there. When I skeptically asked Dr. Dill, "What committee is the right committee?" he answered falteringly, "There is no committee to handle this."

I got the picture. The grievance process had been halted.

I made appointments with Chancellor Krevans and with Dr. Rapaport individually and I talked to them at length.

To Dr. Krevans I said, "You know what has been happening to me. You know there has been a concerted effort to intimidate me. The grievance committee process has come to a halt. I am not going to continue this in any more committees because it takes up too much of my time. I will lose just by being distracted from what I need to do. If you people are successful in distracting me from my purpose of warning health care workers, then you will win. I am not going to let you do that. I am going to continue doing what I have been doing all along—talking about the risks of contracting AIDS through occupational exposure."

I turned to Chancellor Krevans and put my grievance right to his chest, "Do you deny that over the past year the University has attempted to intimidate me over and over again?"

Behind closed doors, here's what he answered: "No, I don't deny it. The interesting thing is that you have been right all along."

Too bad he won't say that publicly.

Shortly thereafter, I was serving as a member on the AIDS Committee at San Francisco General Hospital.

Many of the people on that committee were not professionals with a medical degree but were administrative personnel or persons engaged in assorted auxiliary services. I was the only surgeon on the committee.

I had brought some pictures of surgical procedures along. They were not exactly Ben Casey type pictures. They were bloody trauma pictures taken in a bloody trauma operating room.

When I pulled out my pictures to speak of grave risk in a blood-spattered operating room, Dr. John Luce, a pulmonary doctor (non-surgeon) who was at that time Chief of Staff, startled everyone. John slammed his fist down on the desk, made several papers jump, and shouted, "That does it! That does it! I am sick and tired of this!"

At this outburst, the entire AIDS Committee became wide-eyed.

John yelled at me, "I am sick and tired, Lorraine, of you parading your risk!"

I said, "Parading my risk?"

He shouted, "That's right! Parading your risk! I can't stand this! I am going to walk out!"

Everybody was startled by this outburst.

When the committee meeting ended, Dr. Luce left abruptly, and several shaken AIDS Committee members came and said to me, "We don't know what is wrong with Dr. Luce, but we are thankful that you brought those bloody pictures because now, you see, we think we understand what goes on in the operating room."

A bit shaken myself, I went up to my office, and there was John, outside my office door.

He said, "I have to talk to you."

He came in and sat down. I followed, and I sat down also.

I began, "I don't know, John, what got to you so much during that meeting. Something must be eating on you besides what was going on at that committee meeting. It wasn't my pictures, was it? What is wrong?"

He responded as he had before, "I am just sick and tired of you parading your risk."

I explained, "It's not as if I walk a picket line. I was talking to a hospital AIDS Committee involved with developing plans to prevent risks to health care workers. The committee members need to know what those risks are. They have to understand what surgeons encounter in the operating room."

We talked about some other things.

Then, finally, it suddenly came in a rush—the age-old jealousy between internists and surgeons.

John exclaimed, "There you go again! Surgeons always think they are better than the rest of us. You must have more of everything. More money. More glory. More training. More hours. *And now you even have more risk!*"

I couldn't believe my ears. Petty jealousy clouding a matter of life and death!

I'd certainly like surgeons to have less risk. But the risk is real. And the accurate numbers aren't yet known. Below are a few documented cases:

A Nashville surgeon, Dr. Harold Dennison who died of AIDS in January, 1989, was likely one of the first surgeons known to have acquired the disease occupationally. He is believed to have contracted HIV from blood that splashed into his eye during a surgical procedure several years before. After the incident he developed a corneal infection and subsequently had a corneal transplant that never fully healed.

The diagnosis of AIDS was made just a few weeks before he died.

Dr. Hacib Aoun, a young internist from Johns Hopkins University, contracted the HIV virus several years ago from a puncture with a hematocrit tube containing HIV-positive blood. He has been featured many times in the media as one of the most tragic victims of occupational exposure.

Frequently when he is shown, a drawing of a large laboratory tube is shown. The implication is that he contracted AIDS through rather massive injury such as an inch-long gash.

That is not so. A hematocrit tube has a diameter of several millimeters only—much like the thickness of a pencil lead. It breaks very easily. The wound must have been small and his contamination with HIV-positive blood must have been minimal, but he contracted the disease.

Dr. Veronica Prego, a physician at Kings County Hospital in New York, is believed to have contracted HIV infection when she was stuck seven years ago while picking up tangled gauze and bed linens that contained a bloody needle.

In 1987, Dr. Prego was diagnosed as having AIDS. She sued Kings County Hospital to bring attention to the need for protection. The courts decided recently that she had a valid claim. According to the newspapers, she won a token settlement. She is too sick to contest it.

The cases cited above are, as yet, sporadic and few—but remember in 1981, we only had a few sporadic cases in the homosexual population.

Now we have 83,000 dead and an estimated 1 to 3 million infected.

"A single death is a tragedy," said Joseph Stalin. "A million deaths is a statistic."

In the health care industry, as elsewhere during this epidemic, officials in positions of power have down-played the seriousness of the problem and failed to perform the appropriate studies early. Dr. Merle Sande, Chief of Medicine and an infectious disease specialist at San Francisco General Hospital, wrote in the *New England Journal of Medicine* as recently as four years ago:

> Remarkably consistent current data indicates (sic) that occupational exposure to patients with the AIDS virus does not pose a serious risk to health care workers . . . .One can therefore conclude that caring for AIDS patients, even when there is intense exposure to con-taminated secretions, is not a high risk activity. . . . *Groups whose members are highly unlikely to acquire the virus (i.e., virtually no-risk groups) include health care workers caring for AIDS patients.*[6] (Italics added)

Sadly, his stand has been disproved hundreds of times as far as contamination with blood is concerned. Will this be true a few years hence regarding body fluids other than blood?

What about the nurses' aides handling hundreds of bed pans, day after day and night after night?

What about the restroom cleaning staff?

A good guess is that any Gallup poll today might tell us many people with administrative powers entrusted with the welfare of health care personnel still think that health care workers' risk is low. The result will be unfounded complacency and widening spread of the disease.

Above all, the health care authorities must admit and spread the word among health care workers that the risk of contamination is real. Universal precautions do not guarantee against HIV transmission.

According to one study,[7] during an average operation, 38 percent of surgeons have blood droplets on their eyewear and 2 percent have had direct contact of blood in their eyes. Because mucous membrane exposure can result in HIV infection, adequate protective eyewear should be worn at all times. Goggles are required for proper protection; eyeglasses alone are insufficient. The addition of a full face plastic shield will give added protection from splashing onto the eyes, face or neck.

Surgeons frequently stand in pools of human blood. Breaks in the skin of the feet from fungal infections or blisters are common. In one study, contamination of shoes with blood was found in 32 percent of surgeons. Waterproof footwear should always be worn, but many hospitals do not provide this added protection. Water resistant disposable knee-high boots will additionally decrease the risk of contamination.

Hands and arms must be protected scrupulously. By protecting their hands, health care workers are protecting their lives. The repeated "scrubbing" that must be done before surgery virtually guarantees that the skin of the hands of surgical personnel will be vulnerable.

Protecting eyes, hands and feet are just three common-sense precautions, but anybody familiar with the milieu in the operating room will know that it is anything but simple to have supplies at hand in sizes that fit.

Here comes the AIDSpeak battle cry: Latex gloves!

Latex gloves are the hallmark of universal precautions. The phrase "universal precautions" has such a reassuring ring to it that AIDSpeak has made it part of its arsenal.

Unfortunately, a phrase cannot protect us from the ever-present hazards of needle-sticks, wire cuts and punctures from fragments of fractured bone and sharp objects used during the average operation. It can't protect us from what might pass through those gloves even if there aren't any cuts.

Gloves, along with gowns and masks, have been used in the operating room for many decades, since shortly after microbes were discovered to cause disease. They were intended to protect the patient from contamination by the doctor's or nurse's hands. Now they are being worn to protect the doctor and the nurse from the patient as well. The focus may have shifted, but the gloves, sad to say, are the same.

These gloves are supposed to "protect" the skin of the hands. There is no such thing as "intact skin" with any health care worker who routinely scrubs, handles caustic fluids or cuts and sticks himself with instruments. Injured hands, particularly in operating personnel, are a constant major hazard for HIV infection.

There can be small cuts or abrasions of the skin on any area of the body at any time. When men shave their faces and women shave their legs, the razor blade leaves minor injuries. Both men and women injure their hands at home while using kitchen knives or from paper cuts.

One researcher did a quick and rather rudimentary survey on hands.[8] The hands of 37 members of an operating room staff were examined with a hand-held magnifying glass (x3). Eighty-one percent of the individuals had chapped hands— that is, they had small skin wounds. Eighty-three percent of these individuals claimed that the causative injury had occurred during work. These wounds are a possible port of entry for any blood-borne infection, including AIDS.

Furthermore, all new latex gloves have holes in them!

Researchers from the National Institutes of Health and Georgetown University Hospital examined latex gloves from four manufacturers using scanning electron microscopy and energy dispersive X-ray analysis.

Freeze-fractured sections of all gloves showed open channels 5 microns in diameter that penetrated the entire thickness of the glove. Since the AIDS virus measures 0.1 microns in diameter, it could easily pass through the 5 micron holes in the gloves.[9]

Against needlesticks, latex gloves offer no protection whatsoever. How does one burst a balloon? With a pin or needle. Balloons are made of the same type of material as surgical gloves, and surgical gloves are just as vulnerable to a pin prick.

Other instruments will injure health care workers. Orthopedic surgeons, particularly, are the carpenters of surgery. We operate on bone. We use our power saws and power drills: The operating room is just like a carpenter's shop where we use wires, screws, nails and hammers.

When we are working in a deep wound with broken pieces of bone, those bone fragments are like wood splinters. They will cut through our gloves and into our fingers. Again, it is not because we are clumsy. It's just the nature of our work.

Let's say I do an operation on a spine. In one particular operation the only way I can protect the spinal cord is by putting my finger in the spinal canal to shield the spinal cord while I put wires through the spinal canal. If I don't use my finger, the wire will go right into the spinal cord and possibly paralyze the patient. I cannot use an instrument to push the spinal cord out of the way because I don't have enough differential sensation with an instrument. With an instrument I might put too much pressure on the cord and cause irreparable damage. Since the only way to protect the spinal cord is with my finger when I put the wire through the spinal canal, it frequently punctures my finger after first piercing my glove.

When I am fixing a broken pelvis around the hip joint socket called the acetabulum, the sciatic nerve is in the way. If I am trying to put sharp fragments together, the only way I can protect the sciatic nerve is to use my finger to push the nerve gently out of the way. I do it very softly, very delicately. And still, because I cannot see around corners, I injure my hands on sharp bone fragments.

And that kind of injury can put me in a coffin.

Double-gloving, wearing two sets of gloves, would seem to be the minimal standard for protection, yet even that is not enough. In the Orthopedic Surgery operating rooms at San Francisco General Hospital, we always double-glove and frequently wear sterile fabric gloves between the two latex gloves. Although this layering will not prevent needlesticks and injuries completely, it does give substantially increased protection against cuts and skin contact with contaminated body fluids.

Even the newer latex gloves being manufactured with reinforced fingertips, will not prevent needlesticks altogether. Gloves made of several different materials including Kevlar, the material used in bullet-proof clothing, are now being evaluated for their protection and sensitivity, but they also don't prevent needlesticks or punctures.

One manufacturer has developed a glove with leather reinforced finger-tips to be worn on the surgeon's non-dominant hand to decrease danger from the needle puncturing the finger-tips during suturing. During long surgical procedures, gloves, gowns and boots or shoe covers should be checked for leaks and tears at regular intervals. If necessary set an alarm clock for a reminder to check for contamination at hourly intervals.

Availability and distribution of protective gear are often hit-and-miss propositions, and often we are sabotaged by a system criminally negligent of or maddeningly indifferent to our safety.

For example, I wear size six-and-a-half gloves. I am in the operating room, all scrubbed and the patient is anesthetized on the table when the nurse says to me, "We don't have any size six-and-a-half gloves, Dr. Day. They are on back order. You will have to wear sevens."

Although even sevens are too big for me there are times when I am forced to wear gloves that are two sizes too big and their dangling fingertips get caught on my instruments, increasing my risk as well as my patient's.

On occasion, I have walked out of the operating room, called the administrator and demanded, "I am not going to operate unless you provide gloves in my size!"

"That's all we have. Sevens!" snaps the person in the supply room to the administrator. Neither of them is involved at all in whether I will live or die.

The central supply employee writes on the blackboard in the office, "Out of six-and-a-halfs," and goes home to have a nice evening.

In the meantime I am stuck in the operating room with gloves that don't fit that I now refuse to wear because they are hazardous and put me at increased risk, waiting for someone to search through the warehouse. Sometimes such a search will suddenly yield an entire box of gloves in my size.

"Look at this! We've had them all along!" chirps the administrator attempting to justify inefficient central supply procedures.

I don't care if they are in a box on a back shelf in the warehouse. Unless those gloves are available to me and on my hands, they are no good to me.

This scenario happens regularly in all hospitals where life or death can be a function of back orders.

Because I am a surgeon, I can put up a fuss but a nurse who can't get gloves that fit is not as fortunately situated in our health care hierarchy.

Who exactly is at risk?

Chances are: everyone whose task is to draw blood; everyone whose job is to clean up after an operation; everyone who handles needles; every surgeon doing surgery; and, all those assisting.

The operating room, particularly, is the battleground in the war with the HIV virus in which casualties are not yet recognized much less accounted for in our government statistics.

Instruments that can't be sterilized by heat must be cleaned with extra care since research has shown clearly that dried blood or body fluids protect the virus from sterilization by chemicals.

In one study, needles recently used by drug addicts were tested for HIV.[10] When the needles contained visible blood residue, 20 percent were HIV-positive. If no blood residue was visible, 5.1 percent were positive. These findings confirm that a quantity of blood so minute that it cannot be seen can still harbor an infectious dose of the deadly virus.

It can be stated categorically that America's 6.5 million health care workers all are at risk. This means not just the doctors, nurses, LVNs and nurses' aides, but also the janitors who handle refuse, scrub the floors and dump the cotton wads. They are at serious risk every time they come in unprotected contact with an AIDS patient's blood or other body fluids. They may be at serious risk every time they touch an instrument, a towel, a glass or a pillow used by an infected patient. If that potential risk has not yet been documented that does not mean the danger does not exist.

The government has ignored the safety needs of health care workers to a criminal degree. The protection has been for the infected at the expense of the uninfected. While the US government will spend up to $6,000 on AZT per year per AIDS patient to prolong his life for only a few months, it will not spend one dime for the protection of a worker who takes care of that patient. Billions have been set aside for the development of treatments for AIDS patients, not one red cent has been allocated for health care workers' safety.

When the New York Committee for Occupational Safety

and Health (NYCOSH) submitted a grant application to the Centers for Disease Control for funds to launch a local Teamsters Union training program for their union workers in the health care industry, a CDC grant management officer rejected the application with the comment, "Except for the prostitution industry, AIDS is not an occupational disease—."[11]

Unfortunately, at the Centers for Disease Control, this sentiment presently is the rule and not the exception. To this organization that is supposed to protect the health care workers of America, our lives are apparently as disposable as our latex gloves.

Health care as a profession is waking up, however. Both staff and students at the University of California, San Francisco have criticized hospital administration for ignoring repeated requests over the past year for proper staffing and necessary safety precautions and training. They are requesting 24-hour IV and blood drawing teams, University-paid disability insurance and specialized infectious disease training.

A poll taken by the *San Francisco Interns and Residents' Association*[12] (SFIRA) suggests that over 50 percent of resident physicians have had needlesticks from HIV-infected or high-risk patients.   Based on current estimates of the risk of HIV infection from needlestick exposure, as many as one resident physician per year at the University of California San Francisco may become HIV-positive from occupational exposure, according to Tim Hofer, M.D., Co-chair of the SFIRA. This prediction casts a long shadow.

Recently, I asked the Dean's office at the University of California, San Francisco, since the University demands that I accept the risks inherent in operating on AIDS infected patients, what will happen to me if I became HIV-infected from occupational exposure.

I was told, "You will receive $896 per month until you die, then $2,000 for your burial." That's Workers' Comp. That's my reality.

And that's the reason health care workers have so vigorously resisted mandatory testing. If they contract AIDS in the line of duty, they will be abandoned by the same institutions that forced them to take the risk. Is it any wonder that health care workers are leaving the profession? I resigned my position on July 31, 1990.

For fifteen years I had been a full time faculty member of the University of California San Francisco, but I resigned from my positions as Associate Professor and Vice-Chairman of Orthopedic Surgery at UCSF and Chief of Orthopedic Surgery at San Francisco General Hospital. The Public Health department leaked my resignation letter to members of the press who wrote the usual articles suggesting that I was quitting because of political and University pressure. And as usual, their reports were wrong.

The truth is, political and University pressure doesn't make me run, it increases my resolve to stand firm and fight.

It was in April, 1989, that I first contemplated resigning from my job. Up until that time, between 10 percent and 30 percent of my orthopedic patients were high risk or had AIDS. But during the month of April, 1989, 90 percent of my patients were high risk or had AIDS. And a majority of those patients required operations. Now nearly every needlestick injury was potentially fatal. For the past five or six years, I had been accepting more risk than nearly every other orthopedic surgeon in the country. I have an obligation not only to my patients, but to my children. I have an obligation to stay alive and healthy to raise them. So I quit.

8

Death by Denial

Ten years ago there were only 200 patients diagnosed with AIDS.

Ten years ago? It seems a century ago.

Now there's a holocaust. Predictions are that by the year 2000, some 60 million people in the world will be infected with HIV, and AIDSpeak insists that the only way to stop this world-wide scourge is "education."   That is like saying that chanting "abracadabra" will stop a raging firestorm.

For the sake of illustration, let us assume that fifty-five acres of brushland were burning. Instead of surrrounding and isolating those fifty-five acres and letting the fire burn itself out, we would assign both firemen and victims in the path of the voracious fire to attend seminars about the meritorious use of water.

We would assign them "fire counselors." We would "increase their awareness of fire. . ." by sending previous fire victims to counsel those in the path of the fire about the impending dangers of fire. They would be taught about the proper use of matches and be shown how to drop their still-smoking matches into some water bottles.

We would spend massive public funds on studying the correlation between the dryness of the brush and the percent of chance that additional acres would also catch fire.

We would extrapolate from the number of estimated sparks to the number of fires most likely to start.

We would pontificate on the sad state of our country by showing that there is a relationship between low socio-economics and aversion to following safety precautions.

We would marshall deriding comments about some people's fire phobia if someone dared to speak up and say: "For heavens sake! It's not a phantom! It's a fire! And fire will beget more fire unless somebody puts it out!"

Any number of reasons could be offered to explain why certain people who know the dangers and the need for protection still do not take precautions and eventually end up as victims of AIDS. But that's not the paramount problem right now. The problem at hand is: Where *is* the fire, and how can we best put it out?

In a health care crisis that looks as though it has already sentenced one in every 100 Americans to almost certain death, you don't waste time on correlations. You don't waste time on aiding fire setters so they can set more fires.

You find out where the fire burns.

You surround it. You make sure all sparks are well-contained.

And then you put it out.

According to a television special broadcast out of California's capitol several months ago, 1 to 3 million people in America are now believed to be infected, and 75,000 have died of AIDS. In a press release only eight weeks later, the numbers of dead reported jumped to 83,000.

In that same story, Gail Westrup, a reporter for PULSE, pontificated "Not only (is education) the best prevention—it is the only prevention."

Where did she learn such a banality? And what is there by way of evidence to back up this statement?

The enormity of lackadaisical attitudes regarding the spread of this deadly disease is hard to comprehend and impossible to defend.

In his May 23, 1990, AIDS Quarterly, Peter Jennings of ABC, called it, "the worst epidemic in history." Less than 10 years ago the infection rate was one in roughly 4 million. Now it is estimated to be one in 100. What will America look like ten years from now? Like Zaire?

One-third of Zaire's population is now believed to be infected with HIV. Only twenty-five years ago the disease in that part of the world was practically unknown.

That leaves us some twelve years.

From the best information available to us right now, we can predict that most people who are already infected will die within the next decade. Millions will die of AIDS in America alone. What is it about us that will not let us look those numbers squarely in the eye and ask, "Just what is going on?" AIDSpeak.

Systematic AIDSpeak rhetoric claims that salvation lies in "increasing awareness." Awareness of what?

As commonly assumed, "awareness" means a condom in one hand, a human rights slogan in the other, and in one's heart a fuzzy resolution — not to shoot drugs, and to cut down on partners at risk.

"Education," as presently defined, is not that hard to understand. It is not hard to teach. It is not difficult to learn.

It says, plain and simple, "Use a condom, make sure your partner is not at high risk, and don't share needles when you shoot up with someone."

That's it.

Most people have learned that, by now. Has that stopped the disease?

All of America has been educated quite sufficiently to the meritorious uses of condoms, to the specific risks of anal sex, to the overt and covert dangers of blood contamination through needles, and to the old Depression maxim that the only thing we have to fear is fear itself.

> Philadelphia—"Despite voluminous educational programs and publicity about AIDS, nearly one fourth of 1,329 persons surveyed in Philadelphia are still engaging in high risk behavior, and large numbers of people have misconceptions about the way the disease is spread," a city official reported March 20.
>
> "While the extent of knowledge about AIDS among Philadelphians generally equals or exceeds that of the rest of the country . . . many Philadelphians have yet to change their behavior as a result of AIDS."[1]

That's Philadelphia. It could be most anywhere.

Here is the latest from San Francisco, as reported by a *Washington Post* reporter upon the occasion of the Sixth International Conference on AIDS:

> Gay men are relapsing into unsafe sexual behavior, and other groups at risk for infection by the AIDS virus are ignoring warnings about the dangers of unprotected sex, according to researchers.

This behavior worries many AIDS experts, who fear the failure of safe sex education could exacerbate the already worsening epidemic.

It also has prompted sharp criticism of the approaches taken by federal and local health officials to promote safe sex, which some AIDS experts say have been too timid and too limited.

"To stop AIDS, we are going to have to be more explicit," said Jean McGuire, director of the AIDS Action Council.

Behind that overall picture, researchers said, are several disturbing trends:

Gay and bisexual men under age 30 are twice as likely to engage in unprotected anal sex—the sexual act most likely to transmit the AIDS-causing HIV virus—than older men.

In smaller US cities, gay men practice unprotected sex at rates as much as three times higher than those in larger urban areas.[2]

Sixteen percent of gay and bisexual men who practice safe sex report relapses to unsafe behavior.[3]

Sexually active, heterosexual high school and college students rarely use a condom.[4]

Last summer, I started a folder called "Spread of Epidemic." Here are some headlines from that file.

AIDS Likely to Become No. 1 Killer in Army

Latinas with AIDS: Life Expectancy for Hispanic Women
is a Startling 45 Days after Diagnosis

Puerto Rico Ignoring the Slums Ravaged by Aids

An Heiress' AIDS: Not in the Script

AIDS Cases Up, Possibly Due to Under-Reporting

AIDs Hits 49 in Soviet Hospital

Blacks' AIDS Rate Growing: State Study Forecasts
      Tripling in 3 Years

Key West Officials Fear AIDS May Overwhelm their County

Alarming Spread of AIDS Virus Among Teenagers

New Aids Cases in S.F. Made Big Jump in March

Widespread AIDs Infection Likely, Americans Believe

Surge in AIDS Reports Continues

The Frightening AIDS Toll in New York City

Rapid Emergence of AIDS in Abidjan, Ivory Coast

These headlines, backed up by medical research, are
stating the obvious: the disease is spreading like fire in
brushwood. It is, by now, on every continent, in all classes,
among all ages. The overall pattern is clear. While, in the
Western world, AIDS was allowed to incubate and to explode
within the gay community, drug users, bisexual males and
victims of contaminated transfusions served as bridges to
introduce AIDS into the heterosexual community, and it is
only a matter of time until there will be no gender distinction.

There has been no slowing of the disease. Whatever
education does, it isn't slowing AIDS. We should be long past
focusing our attention on special "high risk" groups alone.

Estimates are that within three years, the number of
Americans killed by AIDS will be five times the number of
U.S. soldiers who died in Vietnam.

Where is the monument?

Recently I found myself on a TV show refuting Michael

Fumento who was promoting his book entitled *The Myth of Heterosexual AIDS*. He actually had collected some 50 pages of statistics bolstering his assertion that AIDS has not become the heterosexual plague that everybody expected it to be.

He makes the point that there are many more diseases that kill numerically at higher rates than AIDS. He feels that AIDS is getting all the attention because it is such a politically handy disease. The media loves hype, says Fumento and the alarmists profit.

I say that just the opposite is true. The virus profits.

And our media has done its best to underplay the threat.

"Education," as we know it, is not our high priority right now. If learning is paramount, then we should learn to fear the virus.

AIDSpeak must stop. We must confront it head-on and defeat it. It is our enemy.

Repeatedly I am asked, "Why would the government lie? Who or what is behind all of this?" The following vignettes show just how difficult it is to directly confront AIDSpeak. It is unpopular to say we should fear AIDS, and those of us who say it end up with our safety, comfort, professional ethics and personal integrity assaulted. Few people dare to say in ways that make a difference that AIDS must be feared as fire must be feared, for it has a momentum of its own. There is no peaceful co-existence with AIDS.

It isn't bigotry we have to fear. We have to fear the virus.

A few months ago, I was invited by the American Cancer Society to address one of their general sessions. Committees planning these large conventions book their speakers extremely carefully. The program is usually printed well in advance, and only under enormous external pressure will a committee change a program.

In this instance, about five weeks before the convention date, I received a call from an officer of the organization saying that they had "decided to remove AIDS from the program." In other words, they cancelled my appearance.

I said to him, "It doesn't matter greatly to me because I have more talks to give than I can handle. This cancellation for Sunday gives me a morning home with my family. But somebody put pressure on you. Is that not so?"

He replied, "I'm just the emissary."

I countered, "No, you are not. You are an officer of the American Cancer Society. Special interest groups forced you to drop me from your program, didn't they?"

He said, "There was some concern about this and that."

"This is a sad day for medicine," I told this man, "because here you are, being held hostage by special interest groups. It's your convention, isn't it? You are so unwilling to have any controversy whatsoever that you will just cave in. You and your committee must realize that you are at least indirectly responsible for loss of life when you do this. Health care workers are not going to hear about the dangers of AIDS and the need to protect themselves."

The caller responded, "I will take that message to my committee."

That made me educate him even more. I continued, "You are a party to this. You keep absolving yourself of all responsibility by saying 'I will give them the message.' That isn't enough. Think for yourself. How can you do this? Here the American Cancer Society is knuckling under to political pressure!"

Then he asked, "You mean there should be some introspection on my part?"

I replied, "Yes, you have the point. You had better think about what you are doing. This is terrible for your organization not to allow both sides to be heard."

He promised to take that to heart.

I went back to finish my breakfast, thinking, "That's how we allow people to die; we let a committee blot out all dissent."

Another confrontation occurred when I spoke to the Republican Women's Association of Newport Beach, which apparently is one of the largest chapters of Republican women in the United States. My presentation was to be in a theater in Newport Beach, and several weeks before I was to give this program, the people who had invited me told me that they had received tremendous pressure from the gay community demanding either that I not be allowed to speak or that they be given equal time for someone from their group.

I said, "Now that's an odd request. Do I ask for equal time wherever they are making their presentations?"

Because of threats of disruption, my hosts decided to bring in plainclothes police nonetheless.

I arrived with some friends and as we drove up to the front of the building, there were homosexual demonstrators waiting and poised to pounce on my message: AIDS is a disease to be feared.

Television cameras were there to record the scene as several gay activists surrounded us and started screaming and yelling at me.

I started to respond, but it was clear they did not want any answers. They just wanted to scream and yell questions so I went on into the building. Security kept them outside until they paid their admission fee, like everybody else. They did pay eventually, came in and sat down in the front several rows on one side.

All during my presentation they were muttering their disapproval and disdain. Intermittently, they would stand up and shout, "That's not true! That is not true!" They would wave placards. They would hiss. They would boo. They would try in any way they could to disrupt my presentation.

I kept my eye on the plainclothesmen in the building, but I did not want to ask them to remove the demonstrators because the television cameras would pick that up and make it look much more important than it was. Therefore I tried to ignore them. The more I ignored them, the angrier they became.

When it was time for questions, one man from the group stood up and started making absurd claims. For instance, he wanted to know why I was stubbornly refusing to operate on AIDS patients or HIV-positive patients.

I told him I had just spent an hour explaining that this was untrue. I had never refused treatment nor would I.

He said, "You have fear. You told us you have fear."

I replied that fear was a proper emotion.

He yelled, "You are in favor of mandatory testing."

I responded, "I am in favor of mandatory testing. I am not doing it, at present because it is against the law, but I am certainly in favor of it."

He replied with something that's not printable. The audience, at that point, started shouting him down. They wanted him to sit down so other people could ask questions.

He turned around and started getting foul-mouthed with the group, screaming and yelling, calling them four-letter words, making obscene gestures, running up and down the aisles. Other activists joined in. I had had enough, so I called security who came and ushered them out. How can they wonder now why there has been a backlash against gays? They invite anger and disdain with their obnoxious, childish and selfish behavior.

I was invited by the Granada Television Network in Manchester, England to do a segment on AIDS from an American surgeon's point of view as part of news coverage of a national AIDS conference then in session in England.

Even before I left to do this show, the producer and assistant producer had talked to me at different times over the telephone for about an hour and a half.

They knew clearly what my stand was on precautionary measures. They knew that I had operated on as many AIDS patients as any surgeon in the United States. I had made sure they understood that I had never refused an operation for a patient who needed one.

And, finally, they knew—because I made sure they knew and would remember—that I had several HIV-positive patients scheduled for operations right now.

My stand, I emphasized, was simple and up front: I wanted clear acknowledgment of health care workers' risks and better protection for health care workers while they took care of AIDS patients.

Before I went on the air, I met with the producers again for several hours to make sure my contribution to the education of the British populace would not be distorted by AIDSpeak. Not only the producer and the assistant producer were there at that meeting, but also the woman moderator who would take her microphone into the audience. The four of us went over all the AIDS issues one more time.

The show was to be live with a studio audience. They had brought in a lot of people from many different places and, as so often happens with these shows, the audience was packed thematically. They had brought in gay men without AIDS, gay men with AIDS, and hemophiliacs with and without AIDS. There was a high official, a woman, from the British Medical Association. They included a woman general surgeon who operates on a lot of AIDS patients and a British orthopedic surgeon who had written the AIDS guidelines for safety for the British Orthopedic Association.

The show was called "Up Front."

I was sitting in a single chair up on the platform, alone. The audience was out in front. The interviewing woman was walking around, Oprah Winfrey-fashion, talking to the crowd and then addressing me.

As the teleprompter came on with the introduction to my part, the talk show hostess said sweetly, "As you know, there has been an AIDS convention going on in Manchester all last week. We have brought in a woman orthopedic surgeon from America *who refuses to operate on AIDS patients*."

At that my jaw dropped . I had just spent hours with these people!

They knew clearly that was *not* where I stood medically and scientifically.

The interviewing woman turned to me and asked me a question. I took a deep breath, calmed myself admirably in front of all of England and said sharply, "Before I respond to your question, I must tell the viewing audience and the audience in the studio that your introduction was completely inaccurate. I have never refused to operate on an AIDS patient who needed an operation, and I have AIDS patients right now scheduled for operations."

I then started talking about what my stand really was: maximizing our understanding of the dangers of AIDS, the inadequacy of protective measures, the need to test rather than guess and the necessity of de-politicizing this disease.

The audience agreed with everything I said.

The woman administrator from the British Medical Association agreed with me.

The hemophiliacs and gay men with AIDS at least didn't argue. Neither did the woman general surgeon nor did the man from the British Orthopedic Association.

No one attacked me. Everybody agreed with me. This mutual accord was of great consternation to the people putting on the program.

When the program was over and we were back in the Reception Room, I went to the woman who was the producer and I asked, "How could you do that? Where is your integrity? You knew clearly that your teleprompter statement was an outright, blatant lie! You did it for nothing more than sensationalism! If you incite the audience like that, you target me for violence. If something happens to me, my blood is on your hands!"

Her flippant answer was, "Well, you had half an hour to explain yourself, didn't you?"

As it happened, the driver who took me back to the airport had picked me up the day before. In between, he had driven home the woman from the British Medical Association.

This driver said to me, "When I was driving her to Edinburgh, she didn't know that I knew you. She told me, 'I was brought in from Edinburgh to argue against this woman.

When I heard what she had to say, there was nothing to argue against. She was totally misrepresented to me by the television station!'"

In the Spring of 1990, I was invited to address the Jewish Conference on Medical Ethics, sharing the program with speakers such as Dr. Norman Shumway. During my introduction, the rabbi in charge told the audience that several weeks before the conference date, the gay activists began an intensive letter writing campaign to all the rabbis in the area demanding that my appearance be cancelled. The gays threatened to picket the conference and disrupt the meetings if they didn't get their way.

But the rabbis stood firm, informing the gay activists that they had no right to manipulate the program of another organization. The rabbis refused to be blackmailed.

These tactics by gay activists occurred again and again as they tracked my speaking engagements, applying similar pressure to every organization or society that invited me to speak. Many organizations resisted, but others, terrified by the threat of being branded as "homophobic bigots," allowed their organizations to be manipulated by the activists' selfish, intimidating theatrics. Too weak to resist, they relinquished control to those who yelled and stomped the loudest.

In 1989, I was asked to speak to a medical conference in Sydney, Australia on the dangers of AIDS to health care workers. After travelling from the U.S. by plane for most of the day and all through the night, I arrived exhausted at the Sydney airport at 7:00 A.M. To my surprise, I was immediately driven to a television station for an interview while wearing the same clothes I had slept in on the plane. At the station I was informed that the government of Australia had issued a 21 page "white paper" against me. Though the "paper" angrily denounced what was purported to be my "stand" on many AIDS issues, it was obvious that the authors had never heard me speak nor had they read anything I had written. The inaccuracies in that paper were numerous. The newspapers interviewed the Australian Secretary of Health and other government officials who referred to me as a scaremonger and accused me of distorting the truth.

AIDS was not dangerous to health care workers, they fumed, and they certainly didn't need me in Australia stirring up trouble.

To suggest that health care workers were at risk from AIDS was irresponsible and homophobic, they continued, and no health care worker in Australia had ever been infected with HIV from occupational exposure.

The television cameras rolled and the journalists crowded around as the controversy over my visit increased. Many interviewers were hostile toward me and my integrity as a physician was frequently attacked. The gay activists picketed my appearances, carrying placards with messages demanding that I get out of their country.

In the middle of my short visit, after I had endured almost continuous public criticism for suggesting that AIDS was an occupational risk to health care workers, a news cast revealed that new information suddenly had appeared, documenting that two Australian nurses had been infected with the AIDS virus from occupational exposure. Apparently the HIV-positive status of at least one of these nurses had been known to health authorities for a number of months, but the information had been kept secret deliberately.

The networks exploded.

On national television, the nurses association demanded that all hospital patients be tested. The Medical Society representative demanded the resignation of the Secretary of Health, arguing that if the government official had known for months about the infected nurses, he had deliberately suppressed the information, and if he truly was unaware that the nurses had been infected, he was incompetent. After I returned to the U.S., the public brawl continued for days.

How could a whole government become so distraught over one physician warning the public about the risks of a universally fatal disease?

AIDSpeak had travelled 7,000 miles to Australia. AIDSpeak was encompassing the globe.

Recently I spoke to the Sacramento Medical Society at the request of Dr. Ben Kaufman, the Society president, and incidentally, my friend. A week before my scheduled talk, Dr. Kaufman received a letter from the office of David Roberti, California Senate President pro tem, one of the most powerful politicians in the California Senate, registering displeasure at the Medical Society's decision to invite me to speak. The letter intimated that I was spreading gross misinformation about many aspects of the AIDS epidemic. The author of the letter, Stan Hadden, a longtime assistant to Senator Roberti, was, a few weeks later, featured in a Sacramento newspaper story as a gay man with AIDS, who was now too sick to continue on Roberti's Senatorial Staff.

When Dr. Kaufman received the letter he felt it was improper, even outrageous, for a Senator's office to apply political pressure to a medical society. A letter from Dr. Kaufman was sent to Senator Roberti demanding to know if he endorsed this type of political manipulation by his staff.

But before that letter was sent, Dr. Kaufman spoke with Mr. Hadden by phone and asked:

"Have you ever heard Dr. Day speak?"

"No"

"Do you know what she says about AIDS?"

"No"

"Have you ever read anything she has written?"

"No"

"Do you know that she has operated on as many AIDS patients as any surgeon in the country?"

"No"

"Then, if you don't know anything about her, why are you protesting her appearance before the Sacramento Medical Society?"

Mr. Hadden responded that he had heard from *others* that Dr. Day wasn't saying the "right things" about AIDS.

Four months passed before Senator Roberti replied. But his disappointing reply revealed that he was not interested in true leadership, but only in responding to special interest groups in is constituency.

As another example of how pervasive the suppression of accurate AIDS information has become, I decided to send a classified ad to the *National Enquirer*. As everyone knows, the *National Enquirer* will publish the most outlandish and ridiculous stories with little regard for the facts.

My check for the $220 fee required to run a 1/2 inch classified ad was enclosed with my ad copy. The ad read:

"If you think the government isn't telling you the whole truth about AIDS, you're right! For free information compiled from the most respected medical journals, by an internationally known surgeon, send a self-addressed stamped enveloped to. . ." and I included the address.

Then I waited for the ad to appear.

The *National Enquirer* requires that all who advertise in their publication must send their product with their ad for approval by the staff to "protect our customers" from fraudulent advertising.   I compiled and sent to them, two pages of summaries of AIDS articles published in the most respected medical journals in the country, such as the *New England Journal of Medicine*, the *Journal of the American Medical Association, and Lancet,* documenting facts about AIDS.

Several weeks later I received from the *National Enquirer* an envelope containing my check, my ad and my journal article summaries with a terse note stating that my subject matter. . .was unacceptable.

Unacceptable? For the *National Enquirer*? Unbelievable.

In April of 1991, an article appeared in the *Los Angeles Times* chronicling my efforts to warn the public about AIDS. The following week I received a call from an assistant producer in Los Angeles who works for a major television movie company that has produced some very fine movies.

The woman assistant producer who called me had become interested in the AIDS problem because a friend of hers, a medical student, had sustained a needlestick injury while delivering the baby of a woman whose husband had AIDS. The medical student, naturally was extremely concerned about his injury, and requested that the patient agree to an AIDS test. She refused, and California law protected both her right to confidentiality and her right to refuse testing. The medical student had no rights, not even the right to know if he had been infected with a fatal disease. His girlfriend was devastated and frightened about his exposure and potential infection and her own as well.

I was invited to their offices to discuss the possible production of a movie with the story line highlighting occupational risks to health care workers, the necessity for AIDS testing of patients and doctors and the resistance I had encountered during the years I had been speaking out on these issues.

"Why," the assistant producer asked during our conversation, "can't my friend demand that his patient be tested? Why must he be forced to endure the mental suffering of not knowing whether he might be infected? What does he do about his life? What does he do about his relationship with his girlfriend? Why doesn't he have the right to know?"

We discussed the reasons for the unfair laws that give no rights to health care workers, the medical establishment's lack of courage in addressing these issues and the tremendous pressure from the gay community from activists inside and outside the medical associations.

By that time another producer had joined us, one who was higher on the decision-making pyramid. She was in favor of such a movie.

Rubbing her hands together with great relish, the producer grinned. "This will be great. We'll make a movie that will smear the medical establishment showing that they've done nothing to protect health care workers."

"Wait a minute," I responded, "I admit that the medical establishment has obstructed the control of this epidemic and has misinformed both health care workers and the public about their risks, but the medical organizations aren't the only culprits. You must expose the enormous pressure from gay activists who suppress this information for their own selfish interests. They don't want the public to understand how their lifestyle and especially their sexual behavior in the bathhouses have been responsible for the explosion of the AIDS epidemic in America."

At that, she turned and looked me squarely in the eyes and in a voice filled with finality, said "We're not touching the gay issues. We won't say anything bad about gays!"

"But you must tell the full story," I responded. "How can you place all the blame on the medical establishment and not even mention the pressure tactics of the gay activists?"

She continued in a resolute, determined voice, "I said, we're not touching the gays. There are too many gays in the business. We would never be able to sell the movie and if we did, no station would show it."

Her response surprised me only a little, considering the massive resistance to the truth I had encountered over the past four years.

This was just another day.

As I collected my papers preparing to leave, I said to both of the women, "I'm sorry, but I can't be involved in the production of a film that won't tell the whole story."

As I neared the door, the woman who had initially invited me to the meeting clapped her right clenched fist into the palm of her left hand and said, "I still want to know why my medical student friend can't test his patient."

I looked at her with both incredulity and resignation, then replied, "Your medical student friend can't test his patient because you, your colleague here and your production company don't have the courage to tell the American public the truth about AIDS."

It is sad but true that many medical associations have

taken the easy way out. For years, the California Medical Association (CMA) has resisted all attempts to introduce responsible public health measures to control the AIDS epidemic. Dr. Laurens White who was president of the CMA in 1988, has denounced me as a fascist, and like a misbehaving schoolboy, has hurled personal insults at me on television programs. What an embarrassment for the California Medical Association to have such an uninformed, uncouth and undisciplined president representing them.

AIDSpeak is winning, because we allow it. The truth is being suppressed throughout society; in the movie industry, in business, in the media, in universities, in medical societies, in medical schools, in hospitals, and at every level of government. Those who speak out not only are ostracized by their fellow workers, but from their superiors they receive threats of firing. For telling the truth about AIDS, some doctors have been threatened with loss of medical licensure, severe bodily harm and even death. No wonder so few are willing to speak out!

"How can gays wield so much power?" everyone asks. Boasts a recent AIDS column in a San Francisco newspaper; Gay activists are the ninth most powerful political action committee in the country. Twenty years ago only 1000 individuals in the U.S. were promoting gay rights. Now there are 7000 *organizations* fighting for gay rights.

The Lone Ranger role is one I do not relish. The point is this: Mixed messages must stop.

We cannot have it both ways. We can't ridicule fear of the virus, send people on guilt trips for fearing the virus, threaten, intimidate and denigrate people who *do* fear it, and then wonder why people don't fear it. Right now most people don't fear AIDS as they should.   They feel it will infect somebody else, not themselves. If they fear it, they feel that they shouldn't.

A recent California poll reveals the ambivalence of the public on AIDS. When asked, "Are you fearful of contracting the AIDS virus?" 23 percent answered, "Yes," and 76 percent answered, "No."   When asked, "Have you changed your behavior as a result of the threat of AIDS?" 15 percent answered, "Yes," and 84 percent answered, "No."

I believe that our government wants to keep it that way. In a shortsighted series of policy statements, the people in charge have let it be known that they do not want the American public to panic.

Barring a more sinister motive, I believe that it is reasonable to assume that our leaders want to keep the population calm about the risks of HIV as a crisis management tactic. However, it is also a cover-up.

We have had our cover-ups before—and to disastrous consequences: Watergate, the Hanford Nuclear leaks, Panama and the Love Canal catastrophe. In all these instances important facts were kept from the people. So it is with AIDS.

On one hand, we are told over and over, "If you are not a promiscuous gay male practicing unsafe sex or a drug addict sharing needles, you will not get this disease."

On the other hand, we are told, "Use condoms at all times, and know the past sexual history of your sexual partners."

The implication is that if you use a condom and you are fairly sure about your partner's history, you will not contract the disease. The AIDSpeak line of "reasoning" is that AIDS is very difficult to get.

If an individual has been told repeatedly that there is no way to get this disease except under high-risk circumstances, that individual will not worry.

She may or may not feel her partner is at risk.

He may or may not use a condom.

And speaking of condoms, they slip; they break; they leak.

In one study done last year, 31 percent of homosexual men who had used a condom during anal intercourse reported at least one incident of condom breakage.

Four of the nation's most popular condom brands permitted the AIDS virus to escape in laboratory tests, prompting researchers to warn users that they should not assume that all condoms work equally well in preventing spread of the disease.

> The tensile strength of condoms suffered drastic losses after only 15 minutes exposure to oil or petroleum base lubricants, including baby oil, petroleum jelly or corn oil at body temperature. . . . Other physical properties—elongation at break, burst pressure and burst volume—showed a similar pattern, with reductions of up to 95 percent from initial values.[5]

Will knowing about safer methods control, slow down or stop the AIDS epidemic? Numerous studies say no, for a variety of reasons.

Although 75 teenagers scored an average of 83 percent on a test of the facts about AIDS, more than two-thirds reported having sex without correct condom usage with partners whose sexual history was unknown.

New York male hustlers were willing to use condoms on male partners, but not with women, one study found. "They know that it's more difficult for a woman to transmit HIV to a man than the other way around, and therefore, the perceived threat to themselves was lower. Also, they perceived their partners to be safe; they don't believe they have AIDS."

In one study in June of last year in San Francisco, nearly half the teens said "sex without condoms is worth the risk of AIDS."

A Canadian survey of white, middle-class college students found that while 80 percent knew condoms were the best protection against HIV and other sexually transmitted diseases, only 19 percent used them.

"Hemophiliac adolescents are not practicing safe sex, despite awareness of the importance of using condoms," according to a recent study.

The study said participants had a high level of knowledge about the cause, transmission and prevention of AIDS. This knowledge, however, was not predictive of behavior with regard to safe sexual practices.

Young and old know about condoms. They know about spermicides. They know about "partners at risk." Yet knowing about condoms and "high risk" doesn't seem to make a difference in behavior.

As one fairly well-educated male put it when asked about the dangers of AIDS and his attitudes regarding keeping himself out of harm's way, "AIDS is pretty much a disease you will have to *want* to have."

This attitude was seconded by a San Francisco teenager who told an interviewer, "I didn't think teenagers could get AIDS."

So what is the solution? More condoms, says the government. The previous Surgeon General has recommended condoms as the main line of defense. A well-known tongue-in-cheek pun urges men to "dress for the occasion."

Some health care workers have been urged to eroticize condoms so as to make them more sexually desirable. The liberal argument is that there should be condom dispensers in high schools. At the very least, the AIDSpeak argument goes, they ought to be handed out free in the streets.

The plain and simple truth is: Condoms aren't safe.

Long before AIDS started ravaging America, women knew that condoms weren't safe. The newest figures on pregnancy show that condoms are just about the most unreliable form of birth control. With the regular use of condoms, 14.2 percent of women will get pregnant[6], even though an ovum is receptive to sperm only three or four days in a month.

AIDS can be transmitted any day of the month.

Common sense would tell you that the rate of transmission for AIDS would be a multiple of the 14.2 percent rate of a potential pregnancy—double, triple or quadruple that figure.

This is not safe sex!

In fact, the government admitted as much. Several years ago, a large grant was given to UCLA for a study using condoms as a method of preventing transmission of HIV from one homosexual man to another.

This grant was withdrawn shortly thereafter because someone from the National Institutes of Health had the courage to stand up and say, "We're withdrawing this money from UCLA because our pilot studies show that condoms are not safe and too many gay men would be at risk of contracting AIDS even during this study."

We do some amazingly fanciful footwork to find out, statistically, over and over, what we already know. For example, we do a study and find out that only a few addicts having sex use condoms. And then we do another study to find out why they don't. We expand our study to suburban teenagers and find out that they don't like to use condoms, either. Then we must study why they don't because we can't extrapolate from addicts to suburban teenagers.

We spend a lot of money studying what common sense would tell us in two seconds: condoms don't feel good.

Or else, we change the labels and define the results as "education."

In this way we can call a previous bathhouse an "education center" and a bathhouse owner a "prevention counselor."

It is wise to reduce your sexual partners. That was wise long before we had word about AIDS. Reducing the numbers of partners to one-third, as Randy Shilts has eloquently argued, does not do anybody any good at all if the epidemic still increases three-fold. The net result in terms of risk reduction is still zero.

Using condoms is better than not using them but condoms don't protect sufficiently. It is foolish and counterproductive to suggest that they do. It is irresponsible of "educators" to suggest to America's youth that they will be safe if they are equipped with a condom.

It is wise and wonderfully responsible to avoid sex with someone who engages in high risk behavior. But how will you know? Most people won't tell. In the heat of passion, it is hard to cool off and confess.

All this Russian roulette business detailed above can be reduced to one very simple abstract rule: Anybody HIV-infected should not now—nor ever again for as long as he or she lives— have sex with a partner not yet infected. But if they do, informed consent and maximum protection should be minimum criteria.

Sex without informed consent with an unsuspecting partner, should be treated legally as assault with intent to kill.

If education efforts would grasp that, then maybe "education" would translate to the imperative of testing.

We are already implementing just such a policy in one of our states, Nevada. Not in Nevada's high schools—as one might think if one assumed that Nevadans properly considered the welfare of their children—but in Nevada's prison population.

All new prison inmates in Nevada will be tested for HIV, and those who test positive will be segregated if they engage in behavior that increases the risk of transmitting the virus, such as battery, sexual intercourse or IV drug abuse.

The new law, AB 186, became effective Oct 1, 1989. It will remain in effect unless AIDSpeak destroys it.

That's one state out of fifty. The forty-nine other states still assign more rights to prisoners with AIDS than to those who are free of the disease. In forty-nine states prisoners have the right not to be tested, the right not to be segregated and the right of confidentiality if they already know that they are positive.

The bottom line is not confidentiality. The bottom line is death.

If our values regarding human rights are so entrenched that we must start by asking poignant questions of prisoners because we cannot bear to ask those questions of our high school students, then let us start with prisoners.

But, what are the rights of *uninfected* prisoners? Few prisoners are under a death sentence when entering prison, although, a death sentence can be easily and swiftly administered to any prisoner by an assault from another prisoner who has AIDS.

Why should prisoners with AIDS have more rights than prisoners without AIDS?

Why should citizens with AIDS have more rights than citizens without AIDS?

Why should the high school student who has AIDS have more rights than the high school student who does not?

Just as prisoners who are uninfected should have the right to remain that way and must have protection from assault by prisoners infected with the AIDS virus, so must your high school son or daughter be protected.

Here is a simple test. The year is 1980. You have one vote to set the course of history. The information you are given is compelling. There are 55 known AIDS-infected people in America. The choice at hand is simple: to use or not to use your common sense. If you decide to use your common sense, then AIDSpeak will not set your policies. If you do not, then AIDSpeak will.

Will AIDSpeak set your policies or will your common sense?

If you decide for common sense, 55 people will be deprived to some degree of what they call their civil rights. Chances are that all of them will suffer as a consequence. Chances are they will not like your common sense at all.

Because they do not like your common sense, they marshal their own troops. They become vociferous. They plot to control your grants, monopolize your media, probe for your own Achilles heel and clutch onto *your* rights to life and liberty by citing constitutional protection for themselves— specifically, *their* right to privacy. The battle gets so hot and heavy that there are times both you and they forget: No one can cure their disease. They will die.

If you don't vote for common sense, they will spread AIDS from coast to coast. In ten short years, an estimated one to three million Americans will be HIV-positive, and 83,000 people in this country will have died. But if your common sense wins, the death toll can be drastically reduced. By how much, we don't know. Nobody knows. One-half? One-fifth? One-tenth?

Would you have cast that vote against your common sense to protect the confidentiality of 55 infected people?

Go to your mirror. Face yourself and ask yourself: Where will this country be ten years from now? Where will your children be?

Had we considered common sense with the fifty-five unfortunate young men first diagnosed in 1980 with an infection linked to the new virus, their suffering might have been compounded by routine health care measures. You would have been accused of infringing on their rights.

Your effort, however, would not have been in vain.

We could not have saved those first fifty-five men. They

would be just as dead. But common-sense measures, prudently used, would have saved many other lives.

Common sense would have set precedents. AIDSpeak would not have consumed us. We could have crippled the virus, and that would have bought us some time.

We wouldn't look like bloody fools today with a leaky condom in one hand, a bumper sticker in the other and a memorial quilt that may eventually cover our country.

9

Is There Any Hope?

September 12, 1988

Lorraine Day, M.D.
Chief, Department of Orthopedic Surgery
San Francisco General Hospital
1001 Potrero Avenue, #3A36
San Francisco, CA 94110

Re: Rumored Prevalence of HIV Positive Blood Donors
at Two Contra Costa High Schools

Dear Dr. Day:

The Alameda-Contra Costa Medical Association
(ACCMA) Blood Bank held a Spring Blood Drive at several
high schools in East Contra Costa last March. There is an
unconfirmed rumor that, at two of the high schools,

approximately 10% of the blood donors were found to be HIV-positive.

If this rumor is true, it would certainly have very strong implications epidemiologically and from a public health point of view. Reportedly, one of the school officials in Antioch who supposedly has this information has refused to comment on it for confidentiality reasons. I doubt that confidentiality applies to statistics when no names are divulged.

Please let me know if you are able to confirm the rumor.

Although I received this letter from an acquaintance two years ago, I have not been able to check out this rumor.

Chances are that two high school principals, with no epidemiological or medical training whatsoever, thinking that their actions are "protecting human rights" are restricting access to data, data which, if properly released to health authorities, verified impartially and acted on responsibly, could well save additional lives.

Again AIDSpeak is costing us. It's costing us in ways both perceived and hidden.

Nothing could be more basic to human rights than the right of the uninfected to remain uninfected. That right *must* supercede the rights of the infected. That fundamental right to remain uninfected can be enhanced by finding out who carries the disease. Unless we know who has the disease, protective measures can't be taken to keep others from getting the disease.

We have taken that approach with every other contagious

disease, whether it is sexually transmitted or not. We do not have to write new rules for AIDS. We have the health care mechanisms locked in place and universally accepted by medicine and lay people alike.

Nobody worries about these rules when applied to syphilis, for example.

Were this disease smallpox rather than AIDS, there would be no shouts of infringement of rights. Nobody would fear political fallout.

Were it tuberculosis, we would not have to argue that infected teachers should not teach and infected health care workers not be around premature babies.

Every reasonable citizen understands that to control a contagious disease, certain rights will be infringed upon. Measures for control are enacted not to hurt the individual; they are instigated to protect society from harm. Such a common-sense measure is enacted when your child is sent home from school with the measles and as a result misses a week of instruction. Such a measure is activated also when all health care workers are mandatorily tested and vaccinated for measles.

We must learn to see AIDS as a contagious disease and not as a test of our "biases" that might need adjustment. We can inspect our biases once we have contained the disease.

HIV is a highly contagious disease involving the exchange of blood and other body fluids. Fear of this disease is appropriate fear. To control this disease by proven methods is the task at hand for modern medicine. To pre-empt this virus from public health safeguards for socially faddish reasons is criminally wrong; it is wrong morally, legally, *and* medically.

It is bad medicine.

That is where we should start, by calling it what it is: bad medicine. We must expose unwarranted concessions to special interest groups and make all parties see that long before the sun sets on this virus, there will be hell to pay if the practice of bad medicine continues.

Our legislators cannot write our laws unless they understand that there are costly public consequences to both omission and commission at the expense of the general public, on behalf of special interest groups. From the medical establishment the public must demand strength and integrity in place of situational ethics. The medical establishment must be the source of this strength and integrity. It is as plain as that.

Don't ever say in decades hence you didn't know a holocaust was going on because your government told you that black was white and white was black and you bought into.

It's happening right now. It's happening before your eyes.

More people are being sacrificed right now than were ever sacrificed in Nazi Germany for no better reason than to enhance a minority's political agenda. Exempting this disease from the controls that apply to all other contagious diseases translates into the suffering and death of millions of people who have a right to life, liberty and the pursuit of happiness.

Our public health agencies were set up by your money and my money to track and control contagious diseases and to protect the uninfected. With this disease, it is the other way around. Our agencies protect the infected and sacrifice the uninfected.

AIDSpeak has been relentless in making us believe that anonymity is sacrosanct and of a higher order than safety.

AIDSpeak has made us believe that society has "chosen"

to protect the infected and abandon the uninfected. Nothing could be farther from the truth. There never has been choice. There has been only massive and relentless indoctrination.

"For every credibility gap," said a wisecrack, "there has been a gullibility fill."

The primary reason for this protective attitude toward the infected is that identification of carriers of HIV would implicate "lifestyle." The primary tool for its continuation has been blackmail not against those in that "lifestyle" but *by them* against society in the form of pressure to withhold grants, affect promotions, control access to the media and shameless pandering to constituencies with special interests and hidden agendas. Systematic blood terrorism may well be next on the agenda.

By now, it's moot to state that protecting what many would call an unsavory lifestyle is no longer a valid excuse because the disease is disseminating into non-gay and non-drug using populuations.

In May of 1990, Peter Jennings of ABC stated on an evening news broadcast that worldwide, one in 700 women is believed to be infected by HIV, and the number is expected to triple by the end of the decade. Everyone knows that AIDS is no longer a disease affecting only homosexuals. By protecting their own interests, however, they help keep AIDS from being contained.

These special interest groups have enormous control in manipulating congressional purse strings, in channeling the research funds that go to teaching universities, in exploiting the air waves and the printer's ink—and, hence, in affecting the minds of the people through AIDSpeak.

It's really very basic: testing would demolish closets.

That truth is the brake fluid behind the enormous resistance to testing.

Although testing for this disease has been made to appear unpopular across America, in practice I have found that just the opposite is true: Patients who have nothing to conceal will welcome a test for AIDS with much the same equanimity that they welcome a test for glaucoma.

"But what about jobs?" say the critics. "What about housing? Insurance?"

What about these issues? Let me answer those querries with more questions.

Is it right for insurance companies to pay huge compensation when the policy holder has not been up-front and honest with them? Don't we have to tell the truth when it comes to cancer and other fatal diseases?

Is it fair for the uninfected to share a pool or a jacuzzi with an HIV-positive person when there has been no testing whatsoever indicating that HIV cannot survive in chlorinated water? Many other microbes can survive and the medical literature is full of articles documenting their survival.

Is it right for premature babies with undeveloped immune systems to be exposed to an HIV-infected health care worker because the administrator does not have the authority to make sure that such an individual was screened out? A person passing tuberculosis baccilli would not be employed in the intensive care unit for "preemies."

This is the first disease ever documented in which the individual who has the disease receives all the protection, and those who may be exposed receive no protection—not even notification of exposure and warning about possible contamination. This disease has none of the limits and none of the curbs that control other infectious diseases.

Is this still a free and honorable country if you as a parent do not have the right to find out if a killer disease stalks your youngster? And if the infected youngster's right to an unimpeded education supercedes another youngster's right to life?

Who benefits in the long run except the virus and the undertaker?

In this morning's paper there appeared two small items, buried among crucial things such as horoscopes and community calendar material. Both items spoke volumes to me.

One was an AP release that stated that once again the World Health Organization had "underestimated" the spread of AIDS world-wide.

New projections indicate that 14 million people will be infected in the United States by the year 2002, with the risk of world-wide heterosexual infection increasing. We're talking about millions of lives now as though we're talking about budget deficits. That's what the politicians do. Though it is the individual who has to pay the taxes. In the case of AIDS, that payment comes in tragic installments—one by one by one.

The other little item in my morning mail was an account of just such an individual tragedy—a clipping of a woman's letter to Ann Landers, a woman who found out that her husband had contracted AIDS from a transfusion.

Theirs is a middle class family—two children, two cars and a dog.

What would happen to her? this desperate woman wanted to know. To her children? Her neighborhood? Her marital relations with her husband?

Gushed America's umpire with a readership of many millions:

> Your husband's illness may not be obvious for a long time. As for how your family, friends, and members of the community will react if the word gets out, let's hope that they will be compassionate and kind. . . . AIDS is just another illness.

Ann Landers,
The Stockton Record
June 13, 1990

That's AIDSpeak at its worst.

AIDS is *unlike* any other illness we have known.

This disease keeps itself hidden for years. In the early stages, HIV-infected people look fine, feel fine and have no obvious disease markers that set them apart yet all the while they are lethally infective to others through their blood and other body fluids.

This is the first disease of mankind ever where secrecy is sanctioned, aided and abetted by the government, the medical profession, politicians and the law.

This is the first disease known in medicine in which a doctor does not have the right to know that the patient has the disease.

Virtually all the laws that have been passed relative to AIDS have been written to govern the behavior of those who are *uninfected*. There are *no* laws governing the behavior of those who are *infected*.

Not even syphilis has enjoyed that kind of protection. For years, syphilitic carriers were compelled by law to be tested before a marriage license was granted—wise legislation that benefits the carrier's children and the taxpayer's wallet.

AIDSpeak has managed to set AIDS apart and exempt it from all common sense, all medical safeguards and all jurisdiction. Resistance to finding out the truth about the magnitude of this disease is unparalleled in the history of mankind.

HIV victims have claimed social, legal, moral and medical privileges no disease has ever been able to claim—protection for the infected at the expense of the uninfected. The HIV-infected and infectious who are also, sometimes neurologically impaired, donate blood, fix our meals in restaurants, make love to unsuspecting partners, drive our buses, fly our planes—with none of us any the wiser. We must ask ourselves and not flinch from the answer, "Who benefits?" How much is society willing to pay to buy a few years of anonymity for someone who is doomed, no matter what the rules?

In AIDS we have a disease that is highly contagious through blood exchange and probably contagious through many more body fluid channels than we have been led to believe. From the moment of infection right up to the moment of death—and beyond—an infected victim can pass the virus through his blood and other body fluids. At various stages contagion may be lessened—but we don't know the magnitude of transmission, nor do we know the viral load it takes to cause infection and subsequent death. We do know such a load is very small. A needlestick can do it.

To take wise precautions, we must know more about the temporal progression of the disease and we aren't trying hard enough to learn what that might be. Why is the onset of AIDS very rapid in some and exceedingly slow in others?

At present we also do not know what the viral count is in

different body fluids. Although we know that for blood it is extremely high, it may be negligible in perspiration—but then, it may not be, either. We just don't know. We do know that the virus is present in almost every body fluid; that ought to be enough for us to want to start accumulating more facts.

We have a health care system that at present, is not actively encouraged to ask these simple, basic questions. If someone does, he ususally provokes ridicule.

This is a disease that puts others at great risk from the moment it invades a body to the moment that that body is disposed of—and who is to say that under certain circumstances burial might not cause soil contamination?

How about sewer contamination as the body is embalmed and blood and other body fluids are flushed into buckets and dumped down the drain?

How about contamination into the world of plants and animals and marine life?

Our legal system offers better chances of suing the doctor for trying to find out about a lethal disease than for suing the patient for concealing that disease.

There exists a rumor of two schools where every tenth teenager is said to be infected—and we don't have the popular support, much less the proper medical and legal back-ups, to check out that rumor. What about the more than 15,000 other schools in California? We have no precise count or facts on anything except those who have died.

Some so-called "specialists" sitting in cool offices in tax-supported institutions are supposed to count. While we still can, we must hold them accountable for counting.

We have had deadly infectious diseases before, and we have always counted. In the past, we have kept track of measles, mumps, chickenpox, tuberculosis, and sexually transmitted diseases far less dangerous than AIDS. By both law and precedent, those who may have been exposed have been contacted and told of their exposure.

That's what health care administrators are paid to do.

There's no reason why HIV should be an exception. We must do both contact tracing and follow-up.

How do you do that, though, where there may be hundreds or even thousands of anonymous male homosexual partners in bathhouses, public restrooms and parks for the gratification of one infected individual who thinks it is his "right" to indulge in his sexual "preferences"? Where deadly intercourse takes place without a single word ever being spoken? Where multiple contacts even in one night are the norm and not the exception?

Good question.

What plays into the hands of those with an interest in keeping our public health offices from counting and contact tracing is the nature of this disease itself.

AIDS is a furtive disease. It is almost as if it mimics the closet hiding many of its victims.

By contrast, it is impossible to hide a smallpox infection. If you have pox, your neighbors know that you have pox. If your son has the measles and you send him to school all feverish and spotted, his teacher will send him right back.

AIDS hides and smolders. It takes its time to provoke the body into forming antibodies. Most who are HIV-infected look fine and feel fine for many years after infection. They look like you and me.

Unless we find a readily available test that tests for HIV directly, we can't start counting until many weeks or months after infection has occurred and sometimes the "negative window" time span will be as long as three-and-a-half years. Thus even if we agreed that it is imperative to count and trace contacts, at best the results of such studies would be approximations.

This reality has enormous implications for the safety of the blood supply. It also gives a false sense of security to those who have been tested and told that they are negative. Being told you are negative does not necessarily mean that you will continue to test negative. Chances are that's what it means, but you cannot be sure.

If even though you test negative, and you actually are positive, and you have sexual relations with uninfected partners, you will be putting them at risk. If there is a pregnancy, it may produce a baby doomed at birth.

For most people, it takes more than a decade from infection to the terminal stages of AIDS, but we are not yet sure about the ceiling of the asymptomatic period. From all we know today, the average length is 10 years. Only when the asymptomatic period ends and the patient gets visibly sick, does our government start counting. Finally.

We have never had a disease where proper counting methods have been suppressed by artificial manipulation of its label. With AIDS, that's what is happening.

If a patient has tuberculosis, he has tuberculosis from beginning to end, not just in the final stages. We did not say that polio is polio only when a victim ended up in an iron lung.

We did not argue that it would be discriminatory to identify a polio victim in the initial stages and refer to polio as polio—and, therefore, to prevent discrimination and help this polio patient keep his job, insurance and apartment, we were all going to conspire to find a less incendiary name. With polio, we did not urge the family, much less the victim, to keep the tragedy a secret. With polio, we did not shame the doctor for isolating the patient.

With AIDS, everything is done to keep the numbers down and keep the public from seeing and thinking and speaking out where it counts: at the polls and in the legislature. Powerful political considerations, not medical reasons, explain the appalling undercount of AIDS.

We have been lied to and lied to and lied to. We are being lied to now.

The Big Lie, as far as I am concerned, is that American citizens currently have all the information necessary to protect themselves from AIDS, and if they do not, that's their tough luck.

The party line is that our worry should be focused on three areas: unprotected sex, drugs, and mother-to-child transmission. Said a *Time Magazine* reporter in the wake of the 1990 Sixth International Conference on AIDS, "No one gets it from air, food or water."

But how does this reporter know? He is just repeating a popular notion.

Many previous popular notions have exploded in our faces.

It's not yet ten years since the American people were told AIDS was "just" a homosexual disease.

We were told that women couldn't get it.

We were told that children couldn't get it.

We were told that transfusions couldn't give it to us.

Attempts by physicians like myself to persuade the blood banks to allow patients to donate their own blood were met with vigorous resistance because such a variance meant a change in protocol. Because somebody did not change a protocol, tens of thousands of people have died. As many as 30,000 people may have become infected with the AIDS virus through blood transfusions alone, while those of us who questioned blood as carrier of the disease were smeared as "alarmists."

Originally we were told that heterosexual sex was unlikely to transmit the disease in this country, even though it had been shown to do so in Africa. Although even sixth graders know that, biologically, Americans are not different from Africans, somehow it became a widespread doctrine here that what was happening in Africa could not be duplicated in this country.

This was later shown to be entirely wrong.

Common sense and logic to the contrary, we were told that sex with multiple partners or prostitutes would not increase the risk of AIDS. I am quoting here from a 1987 editorial in a San Francisco newspaper that reflected the public health authorities' consensus at that time.

Entitled *"A Distorted AIDS Study,"* this editorial is critical of a report released by the San Francisco AIDS Foundation which stated that 100,000 heterosexuals in the area could risk catching the fatal disease of AIDS. The editorial stated:

> This report is being interpreted to mean that AIDS is a threat to anyone who engages in casual, male-female sex. That is not true. *There is no scientific evidence to support the study's assumption that the risk of AIDS is linked to the number of heterosexual partners, or even to sex with prostitutes.* (Italics added.)

Of course, this editorial was dead wrong. Now we know

that the risk of AIDS definitely is linked not only to the number of heterosexual partners, but also to sex with prostitutes. Above all, the risk is linked to an increase of victims infected. Where there are more infected people, there will be greater spread. The editorial goes on to say:

> AIDS is spread in Africa through conventional male-female relations. This puzzles researchers, but there is no indication that the disease has or will spread that way in other cultures.

Of course we now know that AIDS can be spread by conventional female-male relations. It happened in Africa. It also happens here.

Needlesticks? Yes.

Kissing? Yes.

Transmission through blood on intact skin? Yes.

Aerosols? Probably.

Contagion through perspiration? Big question mark.

Water, soil, and public restroom toilet seats? Who knows?

We just don't know because research is lacking. Facts do not cease to exist because they are ignored. Now we are older, sadder and wiser.

As late as 1987 we were told that only ten to twenty percent of people who turn HIV-positive would develop AIDS and die. We now know with virtual certainty that anybody carrying the virus is carrying his final script. As judged from the count that we have, most victims are given a decade. These people have been sentenced to a slow, undignified and painful death without the benefit of trial and jury—victims of our appalling ignorance, crusading patronage, social cowardice, pressure politics, medical inertia—and AIDSpeak.

We have a disease that is explosive in terms of both sheer numbers and geographic spread.

It took eight years, from 1981 until 1989, to diagnose 100,000 cases of patients with AIDS in the United States. It will take only a year or two to diagnose the second 100,000 cases.[1] Will it take only weeks to diagnose the third?

Recently the General Accounting Office of the government did a survey in an attempt to establish a more precise number of HIV-infected individuals so that they could plan for future funding for the care of these individuals. They found that the figures from the Centers for Disease Control on the number of HIV-infected in this country had been underestimated by 33 percent.[2]

A recent study, done by Edward Lauman[3] of the University of Chicago, found that the Centers for Disease Control had also underestimated both the number of AIDS cases among whites and the number of cases of AIDS in the Midwest.

A CDC study has shown that 25,000 college students in this country are infected with the Human Immunodeficiency Virus. Multiply that number by four years of dormitory life and you are talking major tragedy.

For the first eight years of this epidemic, officials at the CDC stated that they did not need to know who was HIV-positive in order to control the epidemic.

Never in the history of this country has such an argument been made regarding any other disease. Had anybody counted accurately then, control and containment would have been easier.

In July of 1989, the CDC finally urged that states begin

reporting not only those who have AIDS, but also those who are HIV-infected but have not yet developed symptoms of this disease.

That's almost a decade after the first AIDS cases appeared— after tens of thousands have died and millions are walking around infected.

Although it is still up to the individual states to count, to my knowledge only about half of the fifty are doing reporting and contact tracing.

We must know where we are so that we can assess which way we have to go. We must know more about the transmission characteristics of this disease and the scope of its attack. We must not let the AIDSpeak slogans shout us down. The task at hand is huge. It will take more than my sole voice and this book to make a difference. Here I can only highlight very broadly where we might have to start.

1. We must handle this disease in a medical and not a political way.

Despite the fact that the former Surgeon General has called AIDS this country's number one public health problem, there is no national AIDS plan-of-action, no unifying strategy to curb the epidemic before thousands more die. Medicine must take the driver's seat. It must stop being special interest driven.

No coherent strategy will emerge unless the medical community starts being pro-active rather than reactive. The Presidential Commission on AIDS includes few members with any medical or health care experience, let alone specific expertise related to the AIDS epidemic, and even these people have let us down.

Organized medicine must inform the American people of the magnitude of the risk. Experts agree that a vaccine is unlikely for at least another decade, if ever. AZT may prolong life for a few extra months, but it is not a cure. Furthermore, it has serious side effects and is very expensive. The only way this disease can be controlled is to prevent those who are infected from giving it to those who are not infected.

Therefore, medicine must take a leadership position in terms of prevention rather than damage control. It must do more than crisis management. Medicine must stop being squeamish. AIDS is an epidemic, and epidemics require stringent measures.

We know how previous epidemics have been handled. The government and organized medicine have well-established rules that have been used in all previous epidemics. Other sexually transmitted diseases that did not have this political component were handled without concern about what positivity would mean to the "rights" of the person infected. In fact, syphilis previously was brought under control precisely because patients with this disease were identified, and their contacts were traced. We must do the same with AIDS. If we do not take precautions now, many more lives will be lost.

It makes more sense to stand upstream and prevent people from falling into a river than to stand downstream and try to fish them out. Given our limited resources, prevention of transmission is more efficient, cost-effective, medically sound and ethically defensible than elaborate care of those already infected.

The first objective is to control the epidemic—and in order to do so, we must know who has the disease. We will never be able to control the epidemic without knowing who is infected. Rather than waiting until a large number of people become symptomatic with AIDS, medicine must apply the public health principles regarding control of all contagious diseases to the control of AIDS. The Public Health Departments must *insist* on knowing who has the disease. They must know who is infected so we can start protecting the ones who are not.

A good grip on the numbers, therefore, is essential. To say that we don't need to know who has the disease because we know how it can be transmitted is to say that we don't need to know where the fire is burning because we know how it is set.

Medicine must be prepared to do what is medically correct regardless of political fallout. There is no need to be apologetic regarding the necessity of routine testing. Routine testing is not a new nor difficult-to-implement idea—not even for AIDS. We do routine AIDS testing all the time; we just don't do it in those settings where pressure politics come into play.

Ten million blood donors and two million military recruits have already been tested. If we can test for blood banks and for the military, why can't we do it for our schools? In our hospitals? Why can't we do it for the workplace? When we buy life insurance? Let us decide that we *can* handle the consequences of widespread testing.

Is routine testing expensive? No, not at all compared to what it costs when we don't test. It now costs about $6 for the ELISA, the routine screening test, and $50 for the Western Blot, a test used to verify the few uncertain test results we get from the ELISA. It can cost as much as $100,000 to take care of an AIDS patient from the time he becomes symptomatic until he dies. Thus if 15,000 routine tests prevent even one additional infection through timely contact tracing and notification, the costs of routine testing are cancelled out in monetary terms.

But is the test accurate? The media and the medical establishment have confused the public by repeatedly reporting that there are many false positive and false negative tests with the present antibody tests—yet they tell you that the blood supply is perfectly safe. The same test is used for testing patients and testing the blood supply. The truth is, if both the ELISA and Western Blot tests are used as they should be in all legitimate laboratories, the accuracy is greater than 99.5 percent. If someone has not yet developed antibodies, the test will be false negative. Since the tests are not 100 percent accurate there will be a few false-positives, but there are other tests, not commercially available yet, that can be used to test those few.

Would you suggest that the pint of blood to be given to your injured child in the emergency room not be tested, just because the test was only 99.5 percent accurate instead of 100 percent?

It does not take a genius to see the necessity of testing.

The choice is in sound medicine.

The bonus to society is that practicing sound medicine happens to be cost containment as well.

Public health officials must know not only the size of the epidemic, but also how rapidly it is increasing and whether or not there are new risk groups emerging. The public health system needs these figures to plan for care of the millions of people who will get sick in the future, to provide them with hospital beds and to train a sufficient number of health care workers to treat them.

Medicine must realize that time is of the essence. Up to the present everything that has happened with this disease has happened too late.

And finally, medicine must model the principles it advocates. All health care workers, including dentists, physicians and especially surgeons, must be routinely tested for HIV.

We are now being tested biannually for tuberculosis and routinely for measles. Nobody shouts "Discrimination!" when testing time arrives.

We all recognize it would be highly irresponsible for a measles-bearing health care worker to treat a pregnant woman because contagion might deform her unborn child.

How much more deadly is the same scenario in the case of AIDS.

2. We must revamp our education efforts.

Mixed messages from health authorities must stop. The message must be unambiguous: "This is a big and bad disease and social obligation cuts both ways." Both the infected and the uninfected must learn to act responsibly. Our education efforts should reflect that principle.

Let's say that instead of AIDS we were dealing with smallpox. Imagine a health care system that would inform the population, "Don't forget your condom, and cut down on your partners at risk. If you take precautions, you're probably safe; it's kind of the wave of the future. You can get 'wonderful powers' from association with people with smallpox."

Were this disease smallpox instead of AIDS, we wouldn't have people with smallpox having sex with people who didn't have smallpox. We wouldn't preach, much less write legislation:

"Don't discriminate against people with smallpox. You must let people with smallpox work in nurseries. Just be careful if you have sex with someone with smallpox. Your civil rights allow you to withhold the fact that you have smallpox from your partner, your employer or your insurance company." It would be understood by all how dangerous that kind of recklessness could be. The message would be clear.

Were messages more to the point about the dangers of this disease, our young people would not tell us and each other, as many do now, "Well, shoot, I'm going to go out with this person with smallpox. I'm going to have sex with this person with smallpox. This is a wonderful person because he's got smallpox."

If readers want to argue that smallpox does not equal AIDS because smallpox is more easily transmitted, try substituting syphilis for smallpox in this equation.

A strong message to keep infected people from infecting healthy people must be internalized and acted upon by both the infected and the uninfected.

The infected must be held accountable. They must internalize the grim reality that their infection is for life. A moral obligation comes with that diagnosis.

Being symptom free doesn't mean that an HIV-positive person cannot infect others. The infected must be made aware that never again will intimacy be possible with an uninfected person, even with "protection," without great danger to that person.

We must have public announcements for the infected, "Don't have sex with someone not infected. If you do, you are putting your partner at risk."

Patients with the disease certainly have the right to medical care but along with that right go obligations. The infected must be made to understand that they cannot take medical care and dental care for granted without maximum and willing cooperation to decrease the risk to health care workers— who are, after all, putting their very lives in danger.

Infected Americans must realize that if they have the virus, then they are probably passing the virus. If they are passing the virus, they are causing somebody's death. They are infected from Day One, and they are infectious from Day One. Apparently some stages of infection are more virulent than others, a finding that warrants more investigation. Because we don't have good data on the different stages of viremia and the effectiveness of transmission, that is all the more reason to act fastidiously. All infected victims have the obligation to make sure that they put no other person at risk.

To uphold this obligation we must investigate all possible methods of transmission over the long term and make public pronouncements that accurately and fully reflect the findings.

If blood is in saliva, then blood will transmit through saliva. Let's see what quantity it takes for transmission. Let's see the concentration. Let's not just assume a kiss is safe and broadcast that assumption to others.

Along with the rights of those who are infected, we must protect the rights of those who are uninfected to remain that way. To insure those rights we must have full access to information. The government and the public health authorities, including the Centers for Disease Control, must improve their credibility by disclosing the full facts to the American people. If Americans knew—as at present, most do not, thanks to our "education" efforts—that the virus is present in virtually all body fluids, there would be much more willingness to do what is necessary to keep infected people from passing the disease to others.

3. We must re-think our health care system along sterner, stricter standards.

The great dying has not yet begun.

The symptomless infected who walk our streets today will be in our hospitals tomorrow. Maybe they will be in our streets. Maybe they will lie in your driveway.

Our health care system is simply not equipped to handle what will be the grim reality five or six years from now. We must plan for tomorrow by extrapolating from today—or we can anticipate chaos.

As of right now, there are 500,000 AIDS-infective people in the New York City area alone. It is estimated that in less than half a decade, 50 percent of the hospital beds in New York City will be occupied by AIDS patients. Currently only 5 percent of the hospital beds in New York City are occupied by AIDS patients, and already there is an overload.

In 1986 the amount of money spent treating patients with AIDS and the lost income from patients sick with AIDS amounted to six billion dollars. Estimates indicate that in 1991 that figure will rise to approximately 70 billion dollars. Already burdened facilities will be further stressed. We will be forced to prioritize; we should begin right now.

If as of right now, we could stop all further AIDS infections, we would still have an epidemic of staggering proportions — particularly for Americans who have never before had to face a public health crisis that threatens to cripple the nation's health care system and strip away all sense of decency and compassion for those in need.

To consider such a possibility may seem unfeeling now but will be a necessity tomorrow when all hospitals will have to plan for "allocation of resources." That means using all facilities maximally.

AIDs patients, at present, ask for benefits for themselves at the expense of other patients. At San Francisco General Hospital, the city's only trauma hospital, in the past we would not have allowed a terminal, intubated cancer patient to occupy a bed in the Intensive Care Unit at the expense of trauma patients who could be saved. Yet this happens all the time with patients who have AIDS. A dying patient needs a place to die; he does not need to occupy a place that causes another patient to die. For example, because dying AIDS patients will be occupying so many beds, an eighteen-year-old with a head injury may be forced to go to another hospital where trauma specialists are not available and so might lose his life in transit.

At San Francisco General, we have abandoned established allocation of resources policies. We often have terminal, intubated AIDS patients who are taking up beds in the Intensive Care Unit. These patients are dying, so where they die, as long as there is dignity in their dying, makes little difference—except politically to someone with an AIDS agenda. These dying AIDS patients monopolize our services while someone else whose condition is not terminal is denied space and attention. I have seen as many as 25 percent of our intensive care beds occupied by dying AIDS patients. On the AIDs ward, all AIDS patients have private rooms, while most patients without AIDS must share rooms. We must excercise moderation with regard to special privileges for AIDS patients, or else a public backlash will occur.

I believe that we will have no choice but to restructure our health care system with a view toward special AIDS centers. I believe we will need hospitals and dental clinics across the country designated exclusively for care of patients with AIDS.

That idea, too, is nothing new.

We have a hospital for burn patients in Texas. We have hospitals that specialize in cancer care. In the past we have had tuberculosis sanatoriums. No one has called any of that discrimination.

It is entirely possible that the future will require an entire system of AIDS specialists working in facilities that specialize in AIDS patients' care. In that way, AIDS patients would receive better care as increased information about the disease would be gathered more rapidly and would be available through centralized channels.

Studies have already shown that AIDS patients do better when they are treated in specific hospitals and clinics specializing in their care. To that end AIDS hospitals could be designed with the finest safety equipment and venting systems as well as special protective gear. Training would be targeted so that all employees would know the hazards and safety measures in their working environment and would be assured of maximum protectivion against the HIV virus.

It is proper to note the similarity between the AIDS epidemic and war. Already there have been more deaths from AIDS than from the entire Vietnam conflict. Because of this reality, hazardous duty pay would probably be necessary to entice health care workers to be employed voluntarily in AIDS hospitals.

If it were impossible to staff such hospitals with personnel willing to work in that hazardous environment, then a military-type draft would be necessary. That draft would be short-term. During time of war, certain individuals must be on the front lines taking the greatest risk, but they are not kept there for the entire length of the war. Troops are rotated thus the danger of death to those on the front lines is spread around so that the risk to each individual is minimized. So should it be among drafted health care workers.

4.   We must stop romanticizing AIDS.

Ryan White was probably the most romanticized youngster in the history of any disease. He became an AIDSpeak poster child. Before he died, he was used by the media in a shameless and irresponsible fashion.

We felt for Ryan—who wouldn't? He helped swell a tidal wave of genuine emotions with his sweet personality and courage in the face of certain death.

A Movie-of-the-Week, based on his experience that played several weeks after his death was shallow, dishonest and a disservice to the life of Ryan White. It showed none of the grieving, none of the suffering that happened because of transfusion. The "villains" portrayed in this movie were not the blood banks who had infected Ryan, but a healthy, all-American neighborhood whose natural instincts made it shy away.

The movie ended with an open-armed "enlightened" school accommodating the youngster with an infectious and lethal disease—whereas chances are that same school, might have sent home a child with ring worm, lice or flu.

Smiles filled the screen as the story ended.

The audience felt duly inspired by a truly remarkable all-American boy who did what was right. Right?

What a deadly AIDSpeak message!

The greed of the blood bank that caused this disaster was never once mentioned at all.

We may wish otherwise but showing AIDS in this romanticized way to millions of viewers of one of the most popular daytime talk shows is misleading. In light of what we know already and what we probably will learn tomorrow, what Ryan White believed was wrong. But that wrong information was given to him by sources that he and most Americans have viewed as reliable, at least until now. These sources include, the U.S. Surgeon General, the Centers for Disease Control and organized medicine.

What Ryan believed was graphically expressed in the interview.

Donahue asked Ryan White if AIDS can be transmitted by kissing, hugging or by tears, to which Ryan replied, "Absolutely not." Then Ryan told the viewing audience that even though the AIDS virus is present in saliva and tears, it isn't harmful in such small quantities.

Ryan continued, "Let's say, you know, you'd have to have, like a whole ocean full of saliva just for it to even be a relatively possible chance of you getting it."

As one philosopher has said, "Though millions of people may believe a foolish notion, it is still a foolish notion."

Ryan White was a media child. Before he died, Michael Jackson gave him a car. Phil Donahue, Barbara Bush, Elton John and other celebrities attended his funeral, which was a poignant ending to a courageous struggle.

But what we aren't told is how he died. Chances are his death was agonizing.

When I asked Multi Media Entertainment, the organization that produces the Phil Donahue show, for permission to reprint a 16 line excerpt of the transcript of the Ryan White interview, a common type of request that is granted routinely by virtually every television, newspaper and radio organization as long as credit is given, Multi Media Entertainment, upon learning who was writing the book and in what context it would be used, denied me permission to use the 16 line quotation. Denials of this type are an efficient method of keeping the truth from the public.

AIDS is an ugly, painful and horribly disfiguring disease caused by a virus that does havoc to body and mind before it causes death.

Consider this rather scholastic passage in a newly published book:

> Although the characteristics of the retrovirus (class of virus to which AIDS belongs) predict CNS (Central Nervous System) involvement in AIDS, it nonetheless came as something of a clinical "surprise" that AIDS patients were manifesting early CNS symptomatology. It is now generally conceded that cognitive (thinking and reasoning) impairment is nearly ubiquitous in AIDS patients. In fact, some patients demonstrate signs of cognitive decline in advance of the diagnosis of AIDS. These observations are independent of the presence of opportunistic CNS disease in AIDs patients and have fostered considerable research interest in the neuropsychiatric manifestations of HIV infection, in the pathologic evidence for HIV infection of the brain, and

opportunistic CNS disease in AIDs patients and have fostered considerable research interest in the neuropsychiatric manifestations of HIV infection, in the pathologic evidence for HIV infection of the brain, and in the utilization of CNS diagnostic methods to detect the presence of HIV infectious processes in AIDS patients.

The manifestations associated with CNS HIV disease include early cognitive (forgetfulness, poor concentration, confusion, slowed thinking) and motor symptoms (loss of balance, poor handwriting, leg weakness) as well as depression, fatigue, paranoia, hallucinations, and anergy. Early signs include impaired cognition, moderate to severe psychomotor retardation, ataxia, tremor, paresis, pyramidal tract signs, as well as behavioral signs (apathy, dysphoria, psychosis, regression).

In the later course of the illness, frank dementia is apparent with. . . incontinence, tremor, facial release signs, myoclonus, seizures, and psychosis.[4]

In other words, your mind goes first in a horror chamber prelude to death.

We now take youngsters to the morgue to show them what speeding can do. Maybe we should do likewise to teach our young the aftermath of promiscuity and drugs that leads to AIDS.

AIDS can destroy eyesight as well as impair most other organ functions. It fills up the lungs so that victims will struggle for air as though they were drowning. Many AIDS patients are literally choking to death on the secretions of their lungs.

Some male victims have purplish-black lesions called Kaposi's sarcoma that can occur all over the body but frequently appear on arms, legs and the face. These cancerous growths are undulating, wrinkled, rather heaped-up lesions resembling a relief map and sometimes are as large as an inch and a half in diameter. They can be found right on the end of the nose. Kaposi's sarcoma lesions are seen as the hallmark of AIDS, although now we know that they are not necessarily part of the AIDS syndrome—not all AIDS patients have them, and not all Kaposi's sarcoma victims have AIDS.

Weight loss is always characteristic of AIDS in its terminal stages. A weight loss of up to 70 pounds is not unusual. Many terminal AIDS patients resemble prisoners-of-war; many have the characteristic "AIDS look" which is a "wild-eyed" appearance characteristic of central nervous system damage.

AIDS patients start losing their memory. They have difficulty with the movements of their hands and their legs. They lose their balance and coordination. Some walk around the hospital with oxygen tubes in their noses. Many are dependent on intravenous tubes for many of their medicines. A large percentage lose control of their bowels and bladder and eventually end up in diapers.

The end can be extremely painful.

I saw a man waste away in my hospital—a man who had been employed in a responsible position in that very hospital working with budgets and numbers. He was getting sicker and sicker, but he kept on working, though he was losing more and more weight. At the end his arms were so small that one could take thumb and middle finger and put them around the mid-portion of his upper arm.

Even in this condition he was still working a few hours a week but no one was checking on his mental status during that time.

When he finally was admitted to the hospital, he would stick his hands in his bowl of cereal and try to eat that way. He had difficulty recognizing people whom he had known the week before.

Within a week he was incontinent of bowels and bladder— a man in diapers who was throwing cereal on the floor.

That's the reality. A car from Michael Jackson is the exception.

5. We must look for the virus in places where we haven't looked before.

We have good reason to suspect that HIV can be found where we are told it is not supposed to be but we don't know in what quantity.

If it can be found in almost all body secretions, then common sense would tell us that it could also, under certain circumstances, be transmitted that way. We must research this virus in *all* body fluids; we should have done so yesterday.

Let's pick a target—let's speak of perspiration.

At present I have no knowledge that the virus can or can't be passed through perspiration. Our health authorities don't have that knowledge either.

When I inquired of the Centers for Disease Control about the presence of virus and possible virus transmission through perspiration, there was no information on the subject. None. Since not everybody had AIDS, the glib argument went, then it probably could not be transmitted that way.

We must remember that the same kind of "logic" was used not all that long ago to argue that AIDS was not transmitted by blood transfusion.

It was marshalled angrily to argue against needlesticks.

It is used today to point out that not every doctor who treats the disease contracts the disease.

It is used to refute contagion through kissing.

It is used to tell people that casual contact transmisision cannot occur when we use public restrooms. Skeptics who are talking about possible airborne transmission are sneeringly rebuffed.

But what will we know in a decade?

Because AIDS is a new disease, information about it is constantly changing. This much we know: the experts have been wrong before—many times.

We must have continuing research on possible modes of transmission other than the ones readily acknowledged. We must look at sweat, saliva, tears, urine, feces, nasal secretions and respiratory aerosols produced by coughing and sneezing.

We must look for the virus not just in perspiration and other "direct contact" transmission modes but also in aerosols such as are created by coughing and sneezing or possibly by insect bites.

I know of no published articles that have reported on whether or not the virus has been found in airborne particles created by coughing or sneezing, but that doesn't mean that it is not there. It is entirely possible that respiratory aerosols such as coughing or sneezing do not transmit the AIDS virus—and if they don't, I would be overjoyed. But show me. Show me. And show me again. A very similar animal virus is readily transmitted by respiratory aerosols in sheep, and an AIDS-like disease transmits in horses through horseflies.

Dropping all such studies is premature. We cannot say transmission can't happen if we haven't investigated whether it can or cannot.

We just don't know.

If we don't know, then we must look.

If the virus survives and transmits in minute amounts invisible to the naked eye on discarded needles used by drug addicts, can it then not survive in a mosquito so sated with somebody's blood that it can barely fly?

On languid summer nights we have all squashed mosquitoes on our skin. We know other blood-borne diseases transmit through mosquitoes.

Please note: I am *not* saying here that a mosquito bite can well transmit the virus to an upper middle class octogenarian with neither drug nor sex risks as he is sitting on his balcony.

But, on the other hand, I am not saying that it can't.

More than one species of animals have AIDS-like diseases. We know that the AIDS virus can infect both chimps and Macaque monkeys, though there are species' differences. It is rare for those kinds of diseases to cross between species— but can we rule that out? If AIDS was transmitted from an African monkey to a human to start this epidemic, as some experts believe, why can't it transmit from animal to man again and again?

Where did all these similar diseases come from and why are they so similar? We must at least entertain the possibility that cross-species transmission might occur.

Since we don't know, we must start asking questions. Making a wish list is an appropriate beginning.

We must address potential hazards in non-health care settings.

A fireman who crawls into a burning building in San

Francisco's drug-infested Tenderloin district might need special knee protection to avoid getting stuck with a needle discarded on the floor. A postman emptying a postal box might have to learn not to reach without looking and sifting or to wear heavy gloves—for drug users often throw their needles in mail boxes. These and similar accidents and injuries are known to have happened. How many hazards are, as yet, unrecognized?

Janitors who clean our public restrooms may have to be given more potent disinfectants and more protective equipment and clothing. Hotel workers stripping sheets soiled with blood and semen might have to gown and glove as health care workers do. Or is blood in a hotel room safer than blood in a hospital?

Do we need air ducts out of the AIDS ward into a vaccuum that would treat the air chemically before it would be released? What about a closed air space such as an airplane, for example, where the same air is circulated over and over again?

It is not at all technically difficult to do the appropriate research that will produce answers to these questions. Rather, the challenge in the 90s is to be able to ask appropriate questions without fear of being lynched.

6. We must be sensitized to AIDSpeak in "official" information.

Let me repeat yet one more time, for the record: The brochures that the government sends to our doors inform us falsely that AIDS can be transmitted in only three ways—through the sharing of needles, through sex (particularly anal sex) and from mother to child during birth. (They rarely mention blood transfusions anymore.)

Those instructions are incomplete and misleading. We now know better.

It still transmits through infected blood from our blood banks.

In the health care setting, it transmits occupationally through needlesticks from patient to patient through hospital accidents, from patient to doctor and from doctor to patient.

On the soccer field, it transmits by blood-on-blood in open wounds.

In a traffic accident, it transmits from passenger to passenger.

We are told that casual contact will not transmit the disease—and that is at best a half-truth.

Let's ask for a strict definition of "casual." Does the Centers for Disease Control see a nosebleed as a "casual" contact occurrence? A nosebleed from an HIV-positive person can carry enough virus to kill a medium sized town.

If a poll were taken today, most people would probably state that they don't believe the HIV virus is present in saliva and other body fluids. Their hazy understanding is that it can be found only in blood.

We must have equal access to information that tells us that the virus is in other body fluids and thus may be transmitted in a variety of ways.

The virus can be, and has been, transmitted through kissing.

It can be, and has been, transmitted through occupational exposure—by needlesticks to health care workers.

It can be, and has been, transmitted through intact skin and through non-blood contamination by bodily fluids in relatively small amounts.

It can be, and has been, transmitted from dentist to patient —

at least five times.

We must be given fuller information.

We cannot afford *not* to know.

We must be willing to revise our opinions in light of additional facts. We must learn to tell information from disinformation.

We must discern when special interest groups start filtering the "truth." Off and on you will hear, that the disease has "peaked"—in the San Francisco gay community, for example, "new infections have levelled off sharply."

New infections always "level off sharply" when most people already *have* the disease.

So far, we have seen only the tip of the iceberg of this disease—a disease that is untreatable and 100 percent fatal. Over the past seven years, we have not heard any information about AIDS that has been more optimistic than the information we previously received.

Rather the information has been progressively pessimistic.

Now we know that AIDS can be transmitted through a blood transfusion, and that death can come to a nurse or doctor through a single needlestick, and that patients are at risk from their health care workers.

We know that the blood supply is still unsafe because blood from a certain number of infected donors will not test positive because they haven't had suffecient time to develop antibodies.

Now we know that deep kissing is not safe. Tomorrow we may learn to our great dismay that changing the diapers of an infected baby can be hazardous. We should already suspect it.

No one has ever argued that to fear diseases such as

smallpox or polio was unpatriotic, anti-humanistic and utterly unworthy. Why must those accusations be made of informed people who justifiably fear an unremittingly fatal epidemic?

7. We must take a new look at our anti-discimination laws which currently protect the infected at the expense of the uninfected.

I certainly am not convinced that it is appropriate for people with infectious diseases to be working in food preparation centers, but we are told repeatedly that this is acceptable. Common sense will tell you that a kitchen worker can cut himself while preparing food. Because we still have so little information thanks to widespread reticence of our "experts" to count so as to know, it has been policy that people with AIDS should be allowed to continue working in these jobs. Remember, it is not considered discriminatory when people with tuberculosis are prevented from working in food preparation areas.

Yet tuberculosis is rarely fatal. AIDS is *always* fatal and yet we would not permit a person with tuberculosis to go by whim and preference regarding testing before we let him fix our steaks or wash our salads.

We insist on testing for tuberculosis. We *must* insist on testing for AIDS.

AIDS is *not* just another disease. It is an enormously dangerous disease. As written now the public health laws state that individuals with certain specific contagious diseases should not be allowed to work in certain jobs if they are a hazard to other individuals. All we must do is enforce these laws uniformly.

An HIV-positive person must be assumed to be a hazard to another individual until proven otherwise through basic research. Simple head counts will not do. AIDS patients who are not contagious in their work situation should continue in their jobs—*only* if we have established absolutely that they are not contagious. At this time blanket anti-discrimination laws cannot be justified from a medical perspective.

We also must establish the rate of infection that can occur relative to the stages of the disease. If Stage I and Stages V and VI are highly infective but Stages II, III and IV are not, then it might be hazardous for infected individuals to work at certain jobs during stages of high infectivity.

Is it safe for known AIDS patients to be caring for children in day care centers or to be employed in a senior citizens' home? This is an issue that should be discussed. Young children and elderly people are especially vulnerable to infections. Until we look at all potential methods of transmission, we cannot say that a person with AIDS—and the potential for opportunistic infections such as tuberculosis—should be working in areas such as a hospital nursery that cares for premature babies who have undeveloped immune systems.

We must research those occupations that put certain workers at higher risk, and we must give these workers adequate protective gear.

It may well be that teaching, for example, will be a high-risk occupation in the future—and latex gloves should come with chalk, crayons and pencils. There's not a teacher in the land who doesn't know the drama, excitement and subsequent "spread" of a nosebleed.

It may well be that several years from now being a student will be a high-risk "occupation" also. Youngsters playing contact sports will run into each other and bump into each other—and if a bloody injury results, there could be tragedy. An infected child should not be allowed to play in contact sports because an injury to him could put another child at risk. Golf and tennis are safer.

We know that there is virus in saliva. Common sense would tell us that in settings such as day care centers or in kindergarten, where children are frequently sucking on each other's toys, kissing each other, biting each other, and drooling on each other, there could be potential transmission.

When young children fall down and abrade their knees or cut themselves, they may bleed on other children. That in itself could be very dangerous.

People in charge have to take care of these injuries. They will not wear rubber gloves unless they are told to wear rubber gloves.

The government must tell them. Medicine must tell them. The media must tell them.

Day care center employees also change diapers, and we know that the virus can be present in feces. Rectal mucous membranes do shed blood. This knowledge should be enough to warn those who might be exposed and impell us to provide protection for them.

We know the virus is present in urine, and that children wet their pants. The virus in urine and saliva is in lower concentrations than in blood, but because it's still there, the staff may be at risk.

Much more investigation is necessary before the magnitude of risk is determined for police officers.

Firefighters.

Ambulance drivers.

Optometrists.

Undertakers.

They are all at risk!

They must be protected.

8. We must start asking unpopular questions and make the answers known.

We know that the virus can survive outside the body for as long as fourteen days. Could it be in our swimming pools? Is the chlorine adequate to denature it in large amounts in urine or saliva?

We know that it can survive and remain infective in a dried state for as long as seven days. Can it survive, hence, on the surface of our public telephones?

Can it survive on utensils in a restaurant or on poorly cleaned glasses in a bar? If it does not, can we depend on the gastric juices to kill it? Before it gets into your stomach with its digestive hydrochloric acid, it must pass mucous membranes of your mouth and your esophagus—all of which are packed with Langerhans cells that have HIV-specific receptors. Remember babies have contracted AIDS from mother's milk. How does that happen?

Does this make you squeamish? It should.

Maybe all restaurants and bars need more stringent surveillance of procedures used to sterilize spoons, knives, forks and glasses.

Maybe they will—once their convention business levels off.

The epidemiologists, the CDC and various other health

authorities say that mere suppositions such as I have listed here are simply outrageous because no one has ever been infected through a diaper or a spoon.

But how do they know that it hasn't yet happened? The reality is they simply don't know.

Since they are not testing large numbers of people, it would be very difficult to incriminate a restaurant because it will take years until the virus shows. Currently there is no way to establish direct cause and effect between an AIDS-positive restaurant worker and an outbreak of AIDS a decade later.

There is a way, however, to show cause-and-effect. It is called scientific research. It starts with a scientific question followed by hard and systematic work to prove or disprove it.

9. We need a stronger moral code.

The question, in the final analysis, boils down to this: Are we willing to talk absolutes? Are we talking about allowing a serious decrease of our cherished civil rights?

Yes and no. That is for you to say.

Just as we now withhold a driver's license from those who are too sick to drive, must we withhold a marriage license from infected people to safeguard unborn children?

Since it is now against the law to carry a concealed weapon, might we as reasonable people decide that it will also be against the law to conceal a deadly virus?

We could pass any number of laws that would translate into saving lives but our politicians cannot write the rules unless they have the facts. They must get correct information from the medical establishment. The medical establishment cannot seek shelter behind situational ethics forever.

It seems to me in theory, at least, that stiffer measures are no longer choice; they are, by now, a mandate. My conscience and my training impell me to tell you what I know—and what I know is that *this illness leaves us little leeway.* It gives no second chances. That is an absolute.

In addition to being a doctor, I am a woman . I am a wife. I am a mother. I am a close friend to several gay men. I am an American. I am a product of our culture. I am proud of my own civil rights.

As a realist, I know, that practice in this country will never equal theory. I believe in taking risks only after I have been appraised of all the facts that come with taking those risks. I would not take my risks blindfolded.

If I were HIV-positive, I would not kiss my child. If I had an AIDS-infected child, I would. I would still kiss my child. I would do things with my own dying child that I would recommend other people *not* do just because that child would be so dear to me that I would risk my life.

I would stand in front of my child if someone were going to shoot him but I would not demand that kind of risk taking from anybody else.

If I had other children my risk-taking choices would lessen because my primary responsibility would be to stay alive and healthy to raise the other children. In that case, I would not be in a moral position to take enormous risks for one doomed child at the expense of all my other healthy children. In that case, I would maximize protection. I would do whatever was necessary for the good of the overall family. I would educate myself to the extent I could. I would certainly wear gloves when I touched any of my sick child's body fluids.

Obviously, blanket moral laws regarding AIDS cannot be drawn from a public health stance alone.

As a doctor I can tell you that anal sex with an infected partner is suicide for you. It is murder of somebody else if your sexual needs make you seek out an uninformed and uninfected partner after you have been infected, knowingly or not.

All I can do is warn you. I cannot write the script for you. I can insist, however, on honesty as a prerequisite, and I can draw the line at callous and promiscuous sex.

An HIV-negative person might still decide to have consensual sex with a partner who is infected—but it should be informed consent between two caring, mature, committed adults who share a clear understanding of all risks involved. Consensual sex with ten or sixty partners in one night in a bathhouse slippery with body fluids is in a different league.

It is the individual who violates a safety principle; the public, in most cases, pays the bill.

In our times and in this country, two adult people, after having been apprised of all the risks, including almost certain death, can still decide to put their lives in jeopardy. They have that right. They can stand in the middle of a busy freeway or climb El Capitan or jump off of the Golden Gate Bridge. If that proves something, let them.

They don't have the right to sink the Titanic.

10

We Are At War!

"I'm Mike Wallace."
"I'm Morley Safer."
"I'm Harry Reasoner.
"I'm Ed Bradley."
"I'm Steve Kroft. Those stories and Andy Rooney tonight on 60 Minutes."

Voice-over: The effects of the AIDS epidemic on the health care system are just beginning to be felt. That there's a shortage of hospital beds for people with AIDS is well known. What's not well known is that there may soon be a shortage of doctors and nurses to treat people with AIDS. The plain fact is, one out of five of the teaching hospitals in this country have reported staff members quitting for fear of contracting the virus.

According to Dr. Lorraine Day, respected surgeon and university professor, those fears are justified. For more than a year, she's waged a one-woman crusade warning health care workers about their risks of getting infected, and attacking the medical establishment for underplaying the threat.

This month, Dr. Day became the highest ranking defector, resigning her job as Chief of Orthopedic Surgery at San Francisco General Hospital.

Day: "I'm quitting because the risk is too high to continue to operate on so many patients who are either AIDS infected or HIV infected."

Kroft: "You're afraid of getting AIDS."

Day: "I think that's a legitimate fear."

Voice-over: "Dr. Lorraine Day is so afraid that she dons a space suit every time she operates. It was originally developed to protect the patient from the doctor. Dr. Day wears it to protect herself from the patient—or more specifically, from the patient's blood, which in many hospitals is now considered a toxic substance.

Kroft: "Have you calculated your chances?"

Day: "Someone else described my risk as being twelve percent per year and 49 percent at the end of five years of turning positive from occupational exposure.

Kroft: "A fifty percent chance of getting AIDS

within five years."

Day: "That's what they estimate . . . Why do I have to take care of a patient with a concealed weapon of AIDS and not be allowed to know that that patient has a disease that can kill me, my nurses, and my staff?"

Kroft: "Is it within your rights as a doctor not to perform surgery on a patient that has the AIDS virus?"

Day: "Not at this hospital, because I am in a public hospital. But a doctor who is in private practice has never been forced to operate on any particular individual. A doctor can refuse to take care of a patient if the patient doesn't have any insurance and he doesn't take (uninsured) patients. Why should you force him to take care of a certain disease that he doesn't feel comfortable with?"

Kroft: "What's happened to this notion, this image of the doctor treating plague, treating cholera, treating polio, putting aside self-preservation and self-interest to save his patient?"

Day: "Nowhere in the Hippocratic oath does it say, 'I will commit suicide; I will endanger my life needlessly for the care of my patients.'

"I will endanger my life as long as I have the proper amount of precautions and investigation of my risk. Nobody is doing that.

"That is all I'm asking for surgeons and other health care workers. Help us develop equipment. Acknowledge our risks. Assess our environment. Train us, and help us, and then we are willing to take the risks. But don't throw us to the wolves."

60 Minutes
September 1989 and August 1990

Let's assume you are a lifeguard. You are young and strong, proud and idealistic, practiced and credentialed. You are burning with desire to make this world a better world. You believe with all your heart you have a moral duty to your struggling fellow man.

You are sitting on the bank of a fast-moving river and there is a cliff downstream; there is a gorge. Suddenly, you see somebody floating by who is struggling with the current.

Your instincts surge.

Clearly, a valued member of the human race is in mortal danger of being sucked over the cliff. He has no chance at all. Unless you leap in quickly, albeit at mortal risk to yourself, he is as good as dead.

Training, duty and adrenaline compel you to ignore the peril to yourself as you struggle valiantly to save the drowning victim. The current is violent and the water is cold. There's no one within sight who acknowledges your risk and gives you credit for your struggle.

However, you know what is right. You do the right thing. After all, the better part of living is doing good for others, or so you have always believed.

You are stronger than the destructive forces of nature and

the death throes of your drowning victim who, while struggling to survive, is clutching onto you and pulling you closer and closer to the edge of the treacherous cliff.

You realize his agony now spells the doom for both of you. With superhuman effort, though, you manage to pull him ashore.

You resuscitate him.

Exhausted but proud of yourself, you lean back, out of breath, and you pat yourself on the shoulder.

But what is your obligation to that victim and to society if he jumps up and leaps back in to the river?

That's what gay males and drug addicts have done. They have put us at repeated risk but have refused to take responsibility for putting us at risk. They expect us to be there to "fish them out" by putting our lives right in the middle of the deadly current, and if we resist that, what happens then? We hear about the Hippocratic Oath as though it were the Riot Act.

The Hippocatic Oath says: "First, do no harm."

Nothing in the Hippocratic Oath compels me to do unnecessary harm to my own body. There's nothing in that oath that says that I must risk my life unthinkingly and unnecessarily. And I predict that I am not alone. I am only one of many who will say to this society: "Don't I have rights as well?"

I love the operating room, and I am leaving it. I love it very much indeed, and I will always miss it.

Professionally, it offered me the best: a chance to help society, good training, respect in my community and a sense of strong self-worth. My colleagues were my trusted friends. I'll miss my patients very much. While many of the patients whom I treated were probably life's luckier ones, there can be found in any public hospital the less-than-fortunate folks: drug dealers, hookers, pimps, alcoholics, hard-core criminals. Caring for them was challenging and rewarding.

All that has changed, thanks to a bit of matter so small that two million could crowd on to the period at the end of this sentence alone.

I am putting down my scalpel—not out of protest, as has been so often alleged, but simply because I'm no fool. Nobody forced me out. Nobody made me leave. I left because I will not sacrifice my life just so I can enhance somebody else's political thirst, sexual recklessness or public relations campaign.

One of my friends died of AIDS—a young woman, age 33. I'll call her Joan. She died two years ago in January.

Joan was the outstanding surgery resident in her second year—a beautiful girl, just as sweet as she could be, and extremely capable. A few short years ago, she was working in the pediatric ward and taking care of babies with cytomegalovirus (CMV)—a virus now known to be associated with AIDS. These babies might have had AIDS, but we didn't know it then. Years ago, we had never heard of children who had AIDS—nor women who had AIDS, for that matter.

Sometime after Joan had worked on the pediatric surgery unit, a rumor spread that Joan mysteriously was losing her motivation. She was slowing down and eventually became so listless that it was difficult for her to walk around the block.

In retrospect, of course, we now know that she was getting very sick.

Before long, her illness forced her to leave her surgical residency. Finally, she was diagnosed as having CMV cardiomyopathy, a viral infection of the heart muscle. An illness of this kind was rare in someone so young, but it could happen. We weren't particularly curious about the rarity of her diagnosis though we were very sorry that Joan was so ill.

Because she couldn't tolerate the long hours on her feet required of surgeons in the operating room, she switched to a residency in nuclear medicine. For the next year or two she improved somewhat, but her glow and energy were gone.

About a year and a half before Joan subsequently died, we were all shocked to learn that she had AIDS. That information was like a bolt from blue skies. We were absolutely stunned. AIDS couldn't happen, we thought, to a heterosexual woman, especially not such a vibrant, clean-cut, capable and beautiful woman.

We wondered in a confused and hesitating way, just where did she get AIDS? How could it have happened?

That question also caused concern among risk management officials of the university. Apparently, Joan and her family were convinced that occupational exposure was the causative factor, but her friends were aware that she lived with a charming but somewhat effeminate man who was a part-time actor and a secretary in the temporary typing pool at the university. I remember wondering if he might be bisexual. But Joan seemed very much in love with him and he seemed to be in love with her. Her illness was a mystery. When we learned Joan had AIDS and there was no mistake about that diagnosis, the supposition and consensus were that he had given it to her.

Today I'm not so sure.

I think it is entirely possible that she contracted it from taking care of AIDS-infected babies. Back in those early days surgeons were completely unaware of their risk.

I attended Joan's memorial service held in the Catholic church at the University of San Francisco, and there I sat and mourned.   Had we known AIDS for what it is, we would have offered her protection. Had she known AIDS for what it is, she would not have given her life. It was sheer ignorance on everybody's part that landed her dead in that coffin.

Could Joan have been one of the first tragic cases of occupational exposure? The University, we heard through the grapevine, paid off after her death as though it was just that—occupational exposure.

Her case was never publicized, and AIDSpeak, to this day, keeps our thinking hazy. For several years, she lived with a gay-looking male in what she thought was a monogamous relationship.   I have heard that he died of AIDS also.

Whether she gave it to him, or he gave it to her, is not known.

After her death I kept her picture on my desk as a constant reminder not only of her quiet courage, but of my own continuing risk in the operating room.

I personally know of 17 surgeons who are infected with the AIDS virus from occupational exposure, eight of whom are orthopedic surgeons.

I know of five non-surgeon doctors who are positive from needlesticks, not sustained in the operating room, but from routine patient care on the hospital wards.

For years, they have had no obligation to report to their unsuspecting patients that they could pose enormous hazards. Because they have been tested through anonymous channels, the public health authorities are unaware that these particular doctors are HIV-positive. They haven't told their superiors. Nor will they unless forced to. It is a deep, dark secret.

Why is that so?

In part because of the stigma. In part because the AIDSpeak atmosphere is not allowing them to say what cries out to be said.

As long as AIDSpeak minimizes the occupational risk, we aren't going to know about casualties who will become fatalities. As long as people are afraid that they will lose their jobs and not be compensated fairly or placed where they could do less harm, they will not tell. And these "high risk" professionals, who have continued to practice, have been sanctioned, mind you, by the government and their individual hospitals to keep their infection a secret! Eventually they could pass AIDS on to others.

I believe that the danger from occupational exposure is substantial.

We must know how big it is. We must know where it is. We can't afford to guess.

I *am* afraid. I predict that, as this dread disease is worsening with the stand-by help of AIDSpeak, others will feel as I do, and do as I did. They will leave and go where it's safer.

I predict there will be wholesale flight—not just from this disease within our hospitals and our inner cities, but from our way of life.

This virus has no mind. It has no human rights philosophy. It is a microbe, itself still on the edge of life. It struggles to "survive."

It does so by transmitting and mutating.

As surely as May follows April and night follows day, if it transmits and mutates in ways some of us think it might but many do not acknowledge, the time will come when it will steal your loved one's breath, extinguish your graduate's smile, invade your grandchild's brain.

It can't be left unchecked.

It does not recognize your father's tears, your baby brother's footprints in fresh-fallen snow. It will stop the hum of a lawn mower, the roar of Ferraris, the disc jockey's yelps and the clatter of your mother's dishes in the kitchen.

"Someday I would like to stand on the moon," said one of our foremost astronauts, "looking down through a quarter of a million miles of space and say, 'there certainly is a beautiful earth out tonight.'"

Wouldn't you?

Said Rachel Carson, speaking not of us but of our forests, meadows and oceans in *Silent Spring:* "No witchcraft, no enemy action had silenced the rebirth of new life in this stricken world. The people had done it themselves."

It is a virus. Plain and simple. If we can grasp that much, the battle is more than half-won. It wants to "live." It replicates at a ferocious rate.

In one small drop of HIV-infected blood there lies the potential destruction of all human beings. This virus respects no borders and no boundaries. It respects no democracy, no power, no prayer, no money. It cannot tell the difference between Mother Theresa and Charles Manson. If it gets into yet another body, it will replicate.

I do not claim to have all the answers, not even most of the answers. As of right now, I mostly ask the questions—at risk of being stoned.

Make no mistake, I take with me some bruises. But just the same, as I walk out of my operating room, I take with me the gravity of what is my conviction; that there is the potential that AIDS in all its misery could shatter 1600 Pennsylvania Avenue.

"And what difference," asked Ghandi, "does it make to the dead whether the mad destruction is wrought under the name of totalitarianism or the holy name of liberty or democracy?"

The massive dying has not yet begun.

"In modern war," said Ernest Hemingway, "you will die like a dog for no good reason."

I think there is yet time—but not much time. If it is true that one out of 100 citizens of the United States are now infected, that leaves 99 of us who are not.

Those 99 must say, " We can't afford to hand over all of our rights to the virus and its victims and keep no rights for those of us who have, so far, avoided lethal contamination."

As of right now, we do not have that luxury.

I believe we are at war. It is not yet a civil war but five years from now it could be. I know the virus is an enemy that's ominous. It won't adapt to our rules. We have adopted its rules and they are fiendish rules. Stupid rules. And utterly unnecessary rules.

For we, as educated people, should know better.

I feel anger. Sadness. Dread. But there is more than anger, more than sadness, more than dread—the dismal business of this virus offends me intellectually.

A tiny microbe—a speck that isn't even life or death at this point in its evolutionary path, has found a parasite's existence in our cells—and we? With eons of brain power that came to us at great cost to our ancestry so we can think with logic and precision—how dare we step aside and let self-serving AIDSpeak do our "reasoning" for us?

We may need love, but more than love, we need scientific understanding. Compassion is a "given" in a civilized society when fellow human beings hurt. It's not with love, however, that we build our highways. That's not how we go to the moon. That's not how we are going to conquer a plague the likes of which we haven't seen in some five hundred years.

Said Kirk and Madsen: "Love is an excellent end in itself, but it isn't half so compelling as a means. Over history, love has severed no colonies from their mother countries, nor overthrown any czars, nor obliterated any Nazis, nor produced any civil rights movement. You may discount what the pious tell you, because it is actually rage, not love, that lay behind all these progressive events."

Rage? No.

Just common sense.

Just lots and lots of common sense against the awesome force of nature that will not quit on us because we have some first-rate parlance skills and love to hear ourselves spew forth our AIDSpeak diatribes—cliches and yet more cliches we have let AIDSpeak hatch. Science and reason can kill HIV. A human rights slogan, no matter how ringing, cannot.

"Let us train our minds," said Seneca two thousand years ago, "to desire what the situation demands."

It is a virus. It will replicate. We must surround it and destroy it while we can.

References

CHAPTER 1

1. Gerberding, J.L., et al., Journal of Infectious Diseases, July, 1987, pg. 1.

2. Braathen, L.R., et al., Langerhans Cells as Primary target cells for HIV Infection Lancet, Nov. 7, 1987, pg. 1094.

3. F. Barre-Sinoussi, et al., Resistance of AIDS Virus at Room Temperature, Lancet, Sept. 28, 1985, pg. 721.

4. Morbidity and Mortality Weekly Report, October 7, 1988, pg. 597.

5. Piazza, M., et al., Journal of the American Medical Association Oct. 27, 1989, pg. 2231.

6. Rozenbaum, W., Lancet, June 18, 1988, pg. 1395.

7. Lancet, Sept. 20, 1986, pg. 694.

8. Chitwood, D.D. et al., American Journal of Public Health, Feb. 1990, pg. 150.

9. Hanson, Peter et al., London, St. Stephen's Hospital. Presented at Montreal AIDS Conference, June 1989.

10. Garden, J.M. et al, Journal of the American Medical Association, Feb. 26, 1988, pg. 1199.

CHAPTER 3

1. Schimpf, K., et al., New England Journal of Medicine, Oct. 26, 1989, pg. 1148.

CHAPTER 4

1. Leitmann, S.F., et al., New England Journal of Medicine, Oct. 5, 1989, Vol. 321, No. 14.

2. Cordell, R.R., et al., Experience with 11,916 DesignatedDonors. Transfusion: 1986 Vol. 26, No. 5, pg. 484.

CHAPTER 5

1. After the Ball, Kirk and Madsen, Doubleday, pg. 291-293.

CHAPTER 6

1. Liautaud, B., et al., Archives of Dermatology, Vol.125, May, 1989, pg. 629-632.

2. Lancet, Sept. 20, 1986, pg. 694.

3. Lancet, June 18, 1988, pg. 1395.

4. Lancet, May 5, 1990, pg. 1105.

5. Morbidity and Mortality Weekly Report, May 22, 1987, Vol. 36: pg. 285.

6. Morbidity and Mortality Weekly Report, Oct. 7, 1988, Vol. 37, No. 39, pg. 597.

7. Chiasson, M., Journal of Acquired Immune Deficiency Syndrome, Vol. 3, No. pg. 69.

8. Federal Register (Occupational Safety & Health Administration), May 30, 1989, pg. 23121.

9. Garden, J.M., et al., Journal of the American Medical Association, Feb. 26, 1988, Vol. 259, No. 8, pg. 1199-1202.

10. Johnson, G.K., and Robinson, W.S., Stanford University, Human Immunodeficiency Virus-1 (HIV-1) in the Vapors of Surgical Power Instruments, Journal of Medical Virology, Jan., 1991, pg. 47-50.

11. Braathen, L.R., et al., Langerhans Cells as Primary Target Cells for HIV Infection , Lancet, Nov. 7, 1987, pg. 1094.

12. Federal Register (Occupational Safety and Health Administration), May 30, 1989, pg. 23053.

13. Federal Register (Occupational Safety and Health Administration), May 30, 1989, pg. 23112.

14. Morbidity and Mortality Weekly Report, June 23, 1989, pg. 10.

15. Federal Register (Occupational Safety and Health Administration), May 30, 1989, pg. 23058.

16. Lancet, Sept. 20, 1986, pg. 694.

17. Journal of the American Medical Association, Oct. 27, 1989, Vol. 262, No. 16, pg. 2231.

18. Federal Register (Occupational Safety and Health Administration), May 30, 1989, pg. 23112.

19. Understanding AIDS. A Summary of Surgeon General C. Everett Koop's Report to the American People. October, 1988.

20. Federal Register (Occupational Safety and Health Administration), May 30, 1989, pg. 23118.

21. Morbidity and Mortality Weekly Report, October 7, 1988, pg. 597.

22. Lancet, Sept. 28, 1985, pg. 721.

23. Lancet, June 18, 1988, pg. 1395.

24. Journal of the American Medical Association, Jan 13, 1989, Vol. 261, No. 2, pgs. 244-245.

25. Journal of the American Medical Association, June 9, 1989, pg. 3282

26. Lancet, May 5, 1990, pg. 1105.

27. Morbidity and Mortality Weekly Report, May 22, 1987, 36:285-89.

28. Lancet, Feb. 15, 1986, pgs. 379-380.

29. Hanson, Peter, et al., London, St. Stephen's Hospital.

30. Shelly, W.B. and Juhlin, L. 1976, Langerhans Cells Form a Reticulo-Epithelial Trap for External Contact Allergens, Nature, 261:46.

31. Ramirez, G., Braathen, L.R., et al, In Vitro Infection of Human Epidermal Langerhans Cells With HIV, from Histopathology of the Immune System. Plenium Publishing Corporation, New York, 1989.

32. Braathen, L.R., Presented at American College of Surgeons, Plenary Session, Atlanta, GA, Oct. 15-20, 1988.

33. Friedland, G.H., et al.,New England Journal of Medicine, Feb. 6, 1986, pg. 344.

34. Mann, J.M., et al., Journal of the American Medical Association, Aug. 8, 1986, pg. 721.

35. Morbidity and Mortality Weekly Report, Feb. 9, 1990, pg. 82.

CHAPTER 7

1. Federal Register (Occupational Safety and Health Administration), May 30, 1989, pg. 23070.

2. Hearts and Hulley, Journal of the American Medical Association, 259:2428-2432, 1988.

3. Lorian, Lancet, 2:111, 1988.

4. Morbidity and Mortality Weekly Report, June 23, 1989, Vol. 38 No. S-6, pg. 6.

5. Garden, J.M., et al., Journal of the American Medical Association, Feb. 26, 1988, Vol. 259, No. 8, pgs. 1199-1202.

6. New England Journal of Medicine, Feb. 6, 1986, Vol. 314, No. 6, pg. 380.

7. Mooar, P.A., M.D., Orthopedics Today, June, 1987.

8. Friberg, B., et al. Umea, Sweden, Presented at the International Conference on Blood-Borne Infections in the Work-Place, Aug. 28-30, 1989.

9. Arnold, S.G., et al., Latex Gloves Not Enough to Exclude Viruses. Nature, Vol. 335, Sept.1, 1988, pg.19.

10. Chitwood, D.D., et al., American Journal of Public Health, Feb. 1990, pg. 150.

11. Feb. 16, 1989.

12. Alert and Oriented. Newsletter of the San Francisco Interns and Residents Association (SFIRA), June 1989, pg. 1.

CHAPTER 8

1. AIDS Policy & Law, April 5, 1989, pgs. 5-6.

2. Jones, C.C., et al., Sexually Transmitted Diseases, April-June, 1987, pg. 79.

3. Ekstrand, M., U.C.San Francisco. Presented at Fifth International Conference on AIDS, Montreal, June 1989.

4. Temoshok, L., U.C. San Francisco, Presented at Fifth International Conference on AIDS, Montreal, June 1989.

5. White, N., et al., Nature, Sept. 1, 1988, pg. 19.

6. USA Today, July 13, 1989. Information from Family Planning Perspectives, Alan Guttmacher Institute, N.Y., NY.

CHAPTER 9

1. USA Today, July 27, 1989.

2. San Francisco Examiner, June 9, 1989.

3. Laumann, E.O., et al., Science, June 9, 1989, pg. 1186.

4. Psychological, Neuropsychiatric and Substance Abuse Aspects of AIDS. Editors: Bridge, T.P., Mirsky, A., and Goodwin, F.K.,Vol. 44, Advances in Biochemical Pharmacology. Raven Press, pg. 2.